Nutrition Throughout the Lifecycle

Nutrition Throughout the Lifecycle

Elizabeth Eilender

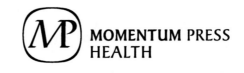

MOMENTUM PRESS, LLC, NEW YORK

Nutrition Throughout the Lifecycle

First published in 2016 by
Momentum Press, LLC
222 East 46th Street, New York, NY 10017
www.momentumpress.net

ISBN-13: 978-1-60650-871-8 (paperback)
ISBN-13: 978-1-60650-872-5 (e-book)

Momentum Press Nutrition and Dietetics Practice Collection

Cover and interior design by Exeter Premedia Services Private Ltd., Chennai, India

First edition: 2016

10 9 8 7 6 5 4 3 2 1

Printed in the United States of America.

To Nicole and Benjamin
Love—M.

Abstract

From birth to old age, there are more than 50 essential nutrients we all require for normal physiological functioning and optimum health. Though everyone requires the same nutrients throughout life, the specific amounts vary depending on age, gender, body composition, health status, and many other environmental and genetic factors.

Nutrition Throughout the Lifecycle provides the reader with an overview of the complex relationship between dietary intake and health promotion and offers students and health care practitioners a detailed reference guide to key nutrient requirements, major food sources, and recommended meal patterns that align with evidence-based government guidelines for adequate intake. In so doing, *Lifecycle* covers the central nutritional issues unique to each major stage of life, including preconception care, pregnancy and fetal development, infancy, early and middle childhood, adolescence, and advanced age.

Adequate nutrition is critical to every stage of the human lifecycle and eating habits during one phase of life can impact well-being and susceptibility to chronic disease in subsequent years. The goal of this book is to summarize the key points and concepts needed to understand the process by which nutrient needs, lifestyle, and environmental considerations affect human health from one stage of life to the next, and how dietary requirements shift with growth, development, and age.

Keywords

adolescence, chronic disease, dietary intake, early and middle childhood, fetal development, food sources, government guidelines, health promotion, infancy, meal patterns, nutrient requirements, older adult, preconception care, pregnancy

Contents

Preface xi

Introduction xiii

Chapter 1   Preconception Nutrition 1

Chapter 2   Nutrition for a Healthy Pregnancy 27

Chapter 3   Feeding the Infant 53

Chapter 4   Early and Middle Childhood 79

Chapter 5   Nutrition for the Adolescent 97

Chapter 6   The Older Adult 121

Additional Resources 149

Index 151

Preface

Nutrition plays a critical role in every stage of life, from supporting the demands of growth and development, to maintaining physical strength and vitality as the body ages. Throughout the lifecycle and for various reasons, people's specific food choices often change dramatically—this is due to a combination of factors such as economics, social pressures, work habits, self-image, health status, living situation, or expanding knowledge about nutrition and diet.

A frail older adult who depends on a caregiver for regular meals experiences eating differently than a person of the same age who is highly active and lives independently. Teenagers are more likely to make food choices based on the opinion of their peers or concerns about weight and appearance, while young or middle-aged couples might be more focused on eating well in preparation for pregnancy.

Though everyone requires the same nutrients for good health, the specific amounts that are necessary for optimal health vary depending upon age, gender, physical activity level, and health condition. From infancy through adolescence, the recommended intakes of macronutrients and many of the micronutrients are higher per pound of body weight compared to those of an adult. Pregnant women need higher amounts of most nutrients compared with nonpregnant women. After these periods of growth are completed, the requirements for calories and certain nutrients decline. Older adults need more of some nutrients and less of others compared to younger adults.

However, chronological age is not always a determinant of energy and nutrient needs, since physical activity, level of relative health, and degree of independence (whether a toddler or a centenarian) all fit into the equation as well.

For these reasons, and many more, *Nutrition Throughout the Lifecycle* is an exploration of evidence-based, applied nutrition concepts. It is intended to offer students and health care practitioners a valuable and detailed overview of how nutrient needs evolve during each major stage of

life, and how environmental, developmental, and psychological considerations, as well as specific disease states, contribute to individual nutrition
status. These days, as the scientific understanding of human health and
disease has grown ever more age-specific and specialized, nutrition, and
public health professionals are in need of expanding resources to keep up
with the recent and applicable research findings relevant to their areas of
interest or practice.

Introduction

At every stage of human development, a regularly balanced and nutritious diet is a prerequisite for a healthy life. In fact, a nutritionally adequate diet is so vital to lifelong health that even the food choices made by mothers during preconception may significantly impact the future health of their offspring decades later. As scientific investigation continues to uncover more insight into the complex relationship between dietary intake and the maintenance of good health, as well as the influence of nutrition on chronic disease development, dietitians and other public health experts must communicate the implications of these scientific findings to an increasingly diverse and multiethnic American population.

Every five years, the U.S. government releases an important set of national guidelines known as *The Dietary Guidelines for Americans*, published jointly by the Secretaries of the U.S. Department of Health and Human Services and the U.S. Department of Agriculture. *The Dietary Guidelines* were first released in 1980 and they aim to provide evidence-based recommendations for diet and physical activity to all healthy Americans aged two years and older. In addition, they provide the bases for designing and implementing health promotion and disease prevention programs at the local, state, and national levels, including social service agencies, educational institutions, and private organizations.

In keeping with advancing research related to human nutrition and health, the most recent *Dietary Guidelines*, released in 2015, aim to incorporate and emphasize dietary recommendations that support individual diet and behavior change; diminish health disparities across racial and socioeconomic groups; and address the prevention of chronic diseases such as obesity, type 2 diabetes, heart disease, and certain cancers (Dietary Advisory Committee Report 2015b).

In the present and the coming years, these diet-related issues must be an urgent priority for federal health officials and for those working in the field of health promotion and disease prevention. The United States ranks 26th in infant mortality among the 29 Organization for Economic

Co-operation and Development countries. A baby born in the United States is nearly three times as likely to die during its first year as could be the one born in Finland or Japan (National Center for Health Statistics 2014). For this reason, improving the well-being of mothers and infants is an important goal for the United States, which can be accomplished through reducing pregnancy-related complications and increasing access to preconception care.

Almost half of all American adults (117 million people) have one or more preventable chronic diseases, and about two-thirds of the U.S. population (155 million people) are overweight or obese (Dietary Advisory Committee Report 2015a)—a growing public health epidemic that has persisted for more than two decades. Data from 2014 indicate that 36 percent of U.S. adults are obese (National Center for Health Statistics 2015), and among children and teens, 18 percent are obese and 32 percent are overweight (Centers for Disease Control and Prevention 2015). Excess adiposity during childhood is much more likely to carry over into adulthood (Freddman et al. 2005), and individuals who are at a healthy weight are less likely to develop chronic disease risk factors, such as high blood pressure and high cholesterol; develop conditions, such as type 2 diabetes, heart disease, arthritis, and some cancers; to experience complications during pregnancy, and less likely to die at an earlier age (Healthy People 2020a n.d.).

Emerging evidence related to epigenetics indicates that nutrient deficiencies during the preconception, fetal, and early infant phases of life may alter gene expression. Such influences on what is known as *developmental programming* may lead to a greater risk of developing metabolic diseases, such as type 2 diabetes, later in life (Vickers 2014).

Traditionally the *Dietary Guidelines* have targeted the general public, but as more data are collected on the importance of dietary intake before, during, and soon after pregnancy, a federal initiative has been established to develop guidelines and recommendations throughout these critical periods to be incorporated more comprehensively in the 2020 guidelines (Dietary Advisory Committee Report 2015b).

At the other end of the lifecycle continuum, older adults are among the fastest growing age group—as of 2013, the number of U.S. residents aged 65 and older reached 44.7 million. By 2030, the vast majority of them will manage more than one chronic condition such as type 2 diabetes, arthritis, congestive heart failure, and dementia (Healthy People 2020b n.d.). These conditions, coupled with the changing nutrient and dietary needs of the aging body, create a distinct demographic with unique health challenges.

Optimal nutrition is vital to every stage of the human lifecycle as one phase of life can predetermine the level of well-being one experiences at the next phase. The goal of this book is to summarize the key points and concepts needed to understand how nutrient needs impact human health and how their requirements change with growth, development, and age.

This book begins by exploring preconception nutrition and moves on to cover pregnancy, lactation, and then nutrition for infants, toddlers, school-aged children, adolescents, and older adults. Each chapter addresses how nutrient needs significantly vary between these major stages of life and explains the impact of dietary intake on the promotion of health and well-being throughout the life span.

References

Centers for Disease Control and Prevention. August 2015. "Childhood Obesity Facts." www.cdc.gov/healthyschools/obesity/facts.htm

Dietary Advisory Committee Report. 2015a. "Scientific Report of the 2015 Dietary Guidelines Advisory Committee: Part A. Executive Summary." www.health.gov/dietaryguidelines/2015-scientific-report/02-executive-summary.asp (accessed June 14, 2015).

Dietary Advisory Committee Report. 2015b. "Scientific Report of the 2015 Dietary Guidelines Advisory Committee: Part B. Chapter 1: Introduction." www.health.gov/dietaryguidelines/2015-scientific-report/03-introduction.asp (accessed June 14, 2015).

Freddman, D.S., L.K. Khan, M.K. Serdula, W.H. Dietz, S.R. Srinivasan, and G.S. Berenson. 2005. "The Relation of Childhood BMI to Adult Adiposity: the Bogalusa Heart Study." *Pediatrics* 115, no. 1, pp. 22–27.

Healthy People 2020a. n.d. "Nutrition and Weight Status." www.healthypeople.gov/2020/topics-objectives/topic/nutrition-and-weight-status (accessed July 7, 2015).

Healthy People 2020b. n.d. "Older Adults." www.healthypeople.gov/2020/topics-objectives/topic/older-adults (accessed July 7, 2015).

National Center for Health Statistics. September 24, 2014. "International Comparisons of Infant Mortality and Related Factors: United States and

Europe, 2010." Centers for Disease Control and Prevention. National Vital Statistics Report, Vol. 63, no. 5. www.cdc.gov/nchs/data/nvsr/nvsr63/nvsr63_05.pdf (accessed June 14, 2015).

National Center for Health Statistics. November 20, 2015. "Prevalence of Obesity Among Adults and Youth: United States, 2011–2014." www.cdc.gov/nchs/data/databriefs/db219.pdf

Vickers, M.H. 2014. "Early Life Nutrition, Epigenetics and Programming of Later Life Disease." *Nutrients* 6, no. 6, pp. 2165–78.

CHAPTER 1

Preconception Nutrition

Introduction

During their reproductive years, women often assume that achieving and maintaining good health prior to conception will likely result in the birth of a healthy baby. This assumption is correct; however, in recent years, we have learned in more detail what specifically characterizes optimal pre-pregnancy health in the months leading up to **conception**, and in the early weeks of **gestation** that follow.

Successful human reproduction involves an enormously complex interplay among genetic, biological, and environmental variables. But when any one or all of these elements is disrupted, such as altered **gene expression**, severe maternal undernutrition, or exposure to high levels of alcohol, fetal growth and development may be seriously compromised.

Popular beliefs about nutrition during pregnancy include the idea that a poor diet is the biggest threat to the proper growth and development of the **fetus**. However, based on recent scientific research, we now know that the connection between maternal, and even paternal, dietary intake and health status even before pregnancy has a significant impact on the health of the newborn, including a risk for chronic disease later in life (Linabery et al. 2014). This chapter explores the influence of nutritional status prior to pregnancy on both maternal and infant outcomes.

Preparing for Pregnancy

Preconception care is now widely accepted to be a critical component of preparing for pregnancy. Factors such as adequate maternal reserves of major nutrients and a woman's pre-pregnancy weight significantly contribute to the health of the fetus. Maternal nutritional status at the time of conception heavily influences the growth and development of the

embryo and subsequently the fetus. During embryonic development, most organs form three to seven weeks after a woman's last menstrual period, and therefore at this stage, the developing **placenta** and fetus are most vulnerable to maternal nutrition status. It is during these first few weeks of **implantation** and rapid placental formation when **teratogenic** effects can happen, and typically before a pregnancy has been confirmed.

This window of time is known as the **periconceptional** period that encompasses the period from before conception to early pregnancy. Throughout this time frame, nutritional and other environmental exposures can impact a woman's ability to conceive and affect the future health of the offspring. For this reason, preconception care is an important component of overall health. About half of all pregnancies are unplanned (Dunlop et al. 2008), and millions of women in the United States do not receive adequate levels of preventative or intervention services because of lack of health care coverage, poverty, risky health behaviors, toxic exposures, and chronic conditions (Centers for Disease Control and Prevention n.d.). Therefore, improving the health of women of childbearing age before they conceive is essential. Previous studies have highlighted the benefits of advising all women of reproductive age to receive preconception counseling on appropriate medical care and behavior to optimize pregnancy outcomes (Dean et al. 2014).

To that end, Healthy People 2020, part of the federal government's national agenda to identify health priorities and improve the nation's health, is presenting a shift in focus from treating diseases to preventing them. The 2020 initiative offers a renewed emphasis on identifying and reducing health disparities, including goals related to the health of women and children (see Table 1.1). Among the 42 topic areas addressed in Healthy People 2020, 27 include a topic area dedicated to maternal, infant, and child health (National Conference of State Legislatures 2011).

Based on these renewed objectives and areas of focus, there are several factors related to pre-pregnancy care that warrant special attention: maternal weight, nutrient intake, chronic disease management, smoking, and alcohol use (Mumford et al. 2014).

Table 1.1 Healthy People 2020 objectives

Preconception care
Increase the proportion of women of childbearing potential with intake of at least 400 mcg of folic acid from fortified foods or dietary supplements.
Reduce the proportion of women of childbearing potential who have low red blood cell folate concentrations.
Increase the proportion of women delivering a live birth who received preconception care services and practiced key recommended preconception health behaviors.
<ul><li>Increase the proportion of women delivering a live birth who discussed preconception health with a health care worker prior to pregnancy.</li><li>Increase the proportion of women delivering a live birth who took multivitamins/folic acid prior to pregnancy.</li><li>Increase the proportion of women delivering a live birth who did not smoke prior to pregnancy.</li><li>Increase the proportion of women delivering a live birth who did not drink alcohol prior to pregnancy.</li><li>Increase the proportion of women delivering a live birth who had a healthy weight prior to pregnancy.</li><li>Increase the proportion of women delivering a live birth who used contraception to plan pregnancy.</li></ul>

Source: Healthy People 2020 (n.d.).

Weight

Studies show that there is indeed a relationship between maternal pre-pregnancy **body mass index** (BMI) and pregnancy outcomes. If a woman is underweight before becoming pregnant, there is a 32 percent higher risk of **preterm birth** and low birth weight; and the health risks associated with a BMI of less than 18.5 kg/m^2 include maternal nutrient deficiencies, heart irregularities, **osteoporosis**, **amenorrhea**, and **infertility** (Dean et al. 2014).

Meanwhile, maternal pre-pregnancy obesity, defined as a BMI of 30 kg/m^2 or greater, more than doubles the mother's risk for **preeclampsia**, **gestational diabetes** as well as increases the risk for **small-for-gestational-age** newborns. Maternal obesity is a cause for **stillbirths,** and fetal and **neonatal** death. Overweight women are more likely to require a **cesarean delivery** and their newborns have a higher risk of being born with a **neural tube defect** or **congenital** heart problems. Moreover, children of obese women are more likely to be obese themselves, creating a perpetuation of overweight or obesity between generations. Despite the risks, losing weight is not recommended during gestation, and therefore the goal is for overweight and obese women to obtain optimal weight status prior to attempting to conceive (Dean et al. 2014).

Pregestational Diabetes

In the United States, more than 12 percent of women of reproductive age suffer from a chronic medical condition, particularly diabetes, which significantly increases the risk of poor maternal and newborn outcomes (Lassi et al. 2014).

Diabetes during pregnancy is associated with increased risk for miscarriages, stillbirth, **macrosomia**, obstetric complications, intrauterine developmental and growth abnormalities, and birth and neonatal complications. It is also associated with an elevated risk of preeclampsia, preterm labor, caesarian sections, and higher rates of fetal malformation and neural tube defect. While tight control of blood glucose during pregnancy is necessary, counseling, diet modifications, and good glycemic control in the preconception period result in an even greater benefit to maternal and newborn outcomes. Studies show that preconception care gave way to a significant drop in **glycated hemoglobin** (HbA1c) levels during the first trimester of pregnancy, along with a reduction in perinatal death (Lassi et al. 2014). Furthermore, those women who pursue medical care before becoming pregnant and maintain good blood sugar control reduce their risk of having a fetus with major malformations to nearly that of the nondiabetic population (Dunlop et al. 2008).

Maternal Nutrition

Recent research suggests that inadequate levels of maternal nutrients during the crucial period of fetal development has an influence on outcomes via the mechanism of fetal **genetic reprogramming** that predisposes the fetus to chronic illnesses in adulthood. Therefore, a nutritionally balanced diet is important before as well as during pregnancy. Many women of reproductive age in the United States do not maintain a healthy diet, and many do not have the financial or geographic access to high-quality foods. In addition, several studies have shown that most women of reproductive age are not getting enough vitamins A, C, B6, and E, or folic acid, calcium, iron, zinc, and magnesium in their diet, and the need for these nutrients increases significantly during pregnancy. This highlights the importance of encouraging healthy eating behaviors during a woman's childbearing years to optimize her micronutrient reserves (Gardiner et al. 2008).

Multivitamin Supplements

Data in the scientific literature supports the routine use of multivitamins by women of reproductive age to improve their own health as well as maternal and child outcomes. Studies found a significant reduction in the risk of preeclampsia with routine maternal periconceptional multivitamin supplementation, along with lower incidence of congenital abnormalities in newborns (Dean et al. 2014).

Vitamin A

Vitamin A is found both preformed in compounds known as **retinoids** (dietary sources include liver, fish, egg yolks, butter, and fortified milk), and in provitamin (precursor) form in yellow–orange plant pigments known as **carotenoids**. The most commonly known carotenoid is **beta-carotene** found in carrots, sweet potatoes, cantaloupe, spinach, lettuce, tomatoes, and broccoli (Table 1.2).

Adequate amounts of vitamin A are essential for vision and eye health, fetal growth, reproduction, immunity, the integrity of **epithelial** tissue, and normal cell differentiation (the process by which immature cells change in structure and function to become specialized). Vitamin A is fat soluble and therefore crosses the placenta easily and has a long half-life. A very high intake of preformed vitamin A (generally related to the use of dietary supplements or medication) is associated with miscarriage and birth defects and these effects are most likely to occur during the first few months of gestation.

The vitamin A content of food is commonly expressed in μg (micrograms) of retinol activity equivalents (RAE). One RAE is approximately

Table 1.2 Selected food sources of vitamin A

Food	µg RAE per serving	IU per serving[Ψ]	Percent DV*
Sweet potato, baked in skin, 1 whole	1,403	28,058	561
Beef liver, pan fried, 3 oz	6,582	22,175	444
Spinach, frozen, boiled, ½ cup	573	11,458	229
Carrots, raw, ½ cup	459	9,189	184
Pumpkin pie, commercially prepared, 1 piece	488	3,743	249
Cantaloupe, raw, ½ cup	135	2,706	54
Peppers, sweet, red, raw, ½ cup	117	2,332	47
Mango, raw, 1 whole	112	2,240	45
Black-eyed peas (cowpeas), boiled, 1 cup	66	1,305	26
Apricots, dried, sulfured, 10 halves	63	1,261	25
Broccoli, boiled, ½ cup	60	1,208	24
Ice cream, French vanilla, soft serve, 1 cup	278	1,014	20
Cheese, ricotta, part skim, 1 cup	263	945	19
Tomato juice, canned, ¾ cup	42	821	16
Herring, Atlantic, pickled, 3 oz	219	731	15
Ready-to-eat cereal, fortified with 10% of the DV for vitamin A, ¾–1 cup (more heavily fortified cereals might provide more of the DV)	127–149	500	10
Milk, fat-free or skim, with added vitamin A and vitamin D, 1 cup	149	500	10
Baked beans, canned, plain or vegetarian, 1 cup	13	274	5
Egg, hard boiled, 1 large	75	260	5
Summer squash, all varieties, boiled, ½ cup	10	191	4
Salmon, sockeye, cooked, 3 oz	59	176	4
Yogurt, plain, low fat, 1 cup	32	116	2
Pistachio nuts, dry roasted, 1 oz	4	73	1
Tuna, light, canned in oil, drained solids, 3 oz	20	65	1
Chicken, breast meat and skin, roasted, ½ breast	5	18	0

Source: National Institutes of Health Office of Dietary Supplements (2013).

* DV = Daily Value. DVs were developed by the U.S. Food and Drug Administration to help consumers compare the nutrient contents among products within the context of a total daily diet.
Ψ The content of vitamin A is expressed as International Units (IU) on dietary supplement and food labels. 1 µg = 0.3 IU Retinol = 0.6 IU Beta-carotene.

1 µg of retinol and 12 µg of beta-carotene. The recommended dietary allowance of preformed vitamin A is 700 µg RAEs per day for nonpregnant women, with a tolerable upper intake level of 3,000 µg RAEs per day, and 770 µg RAEs for pregnant women (Gardiner et al. 2008).

Folate

Folate is one of the B-complex vitamins and is needed for the synthesis of DNA and is therefore required for normal cell division. Because rapid cell division occurs in the first days and weeks of pregnancy, adequate folate is essential prior to and during pregnancy and has a proven role in reducing the risk of neural tube defects. Legumes, green leafy vegetables, citrus fruits, and juices are all sources of naturally occurring folate; while folic acid, a synthetic compound, is available in enriched breads and cereals, and dietary supplements. The current recommended daily intake for folic acid is 400 µg for women of childbearing age and 600 µg during pregnancy. For women who have had an infant with a neural tube defect, the recommended daily amount is 4,000 µg (Gardiner et al. 2008) (Table 1.3).

Vitamin D

Vitamin D is a fat-soluble vitamin that is important in the metabolism of calcium and phosphorous, and promotes calcium absorption and **bone mineralization**. It can be obtained from either bodily production from sun exposure or dietary sources, such as fortified milk, orange juice, and some breakfast cereals. Other dietary sources include fatty fish (salmon, mackerel, tuna, sardine), egg yolks, beef liver, and cheese made with fortified milk (Table 1.4).

Calcium and phosphorous are needed for the developing skeleton of the fetus, and vitamin D is required for the proper absorption and use of these minerals; therefore, it is essential for the health of pregnant women and their infants. Currently, there is an increasing prevalence of vitamin D insufficiency and deficiency in pregnant women and infants in the United States. Women who have adequate exposure to sunlight likely do not need additional vitamin D. However, women who are at risk for vitamin D deficiency include those who are not exposed to enough

Table 1.3 Selected food sources of folate and folic acid

Food	µg DFE per serving[Ψ]	Percent DV*
Beef liver, braised, 3 oz	215	54
Spinach, boiled, ½ cup	131	33
Black-eyed peas (cowpeas), boiled, ½ cup	105	26
Breakfast cereals, fortified with 25% of the DV	100	25
Rice, white, medium-grain, cooked, ½ cup	90	23
Asparagus, boiled, 4 spears	89	22
Spaghetti, cooked, enriched, ½ cup	83	21
Brussels sprouts, frozen, boiled, ½ cup	78	20
Lettuce, romaine, shredded, 1 cup	64	16
Avocado, raw, sliced, ½ cup	59	15
Spinach, raw, 1 cup	58	15
Broccoli, chopped, frozen, cooked, ½ cup	52	13
Mustard greens, chopped, frozen, boiled, ½ cup	52	13
Green peas, frozen, boiled, ½ cup	47	12
Kidney beans, canned, ½ cup	46	12
Bread, white, 1 slice	43	11
Peanuts, dry roasted, 1 oz	41	10
Wheat germ, 2 tablespoons	40	10
Tomato juice, canned, ¾ cup	36	9
Crab, Dungeness, 3 oz	36	9
Orange juice, ¾ cup	35	9
Turnip greens, frozen, boiled, ½ cup	32	8
Orange, fresh, 1 small	29	7
Papaya, raw, cubed, ½ cup	27	7
Banana, 1 medium	24	6
Yeast, baker's, ¼ teaspoon	23	6
Egg, whole, hard-boiled, 1 large	22	6
Vegetarian baked beans, canned, ½ cup	15	4
Cantaloupe, raw, 1 wedge	14	4
Fish, halibut, cooked, 3 oz	12	3
Milk, 1% fat, 1 cup	12	3
Ground beef, 85% lean, cooked, 3 oz	7	2
Chicken breast, roasted, ½ breast	3	1

Source: National Institutes of Health Office of Dietary Supplements (2012).
* DV = Daily Value. DVs were developed by the U.S. Food and Drug Administration to help consumers compare the nutrient contents among products within the context of a total daily diet.
Ψ Dietary Folate Equivalents.

Table 1.4 Selected food sources of vitamin D

Food	IUs per serving[Ψ]	Percent DV*
Cod liver oil, 1 tablespoon	1,360	340
Swordfish, cooked, 3 oz	566	142
Salmon (sockeye), cooked, 3 oz	447	112
Tuna fish, canned in water, drained, 3 oz	154	39
Orange juice fortified with vitamin D, 1 cup (check product labels, as amount of added vitamin D varies)	137	34
Milk, nonfat, reduced fat, and whole, vitamin D-fortified, 1 cup	115–124	29–31
Yogurt, fortified with 20% of the DV for vitamin D, 6 oz (more heavily fortified yogurts provide more of the DV)	80	20
Margarine, fortified, 1 tablespoon	60	15
Sardines, canned in oil, drained, 2 sardines	46	12
Liver, beef, cooked, 3 oz	42	11
Egg, 1 large (vitamin D is found in yolk)	41	10
Ready-to-eat cereal, fortified with 10% of the DV for vitamin D, 0.75–1 cup (more heavily fortified cereals might provide more of the DV)	40	10
Cheese, Swiss, 1 oz	6	2

Source: National Institutes of Health Office of Dietary Supplements (2014).
* DV = Daily Value. DVs were developed by the U.S. Food and Drug Administration to help consumers compare the nutrient contents among products within the context of a total daily diet.
Ψ The content of vitamin D is expressed as International Units (IU) on dietary supplement and food labels. 1 µg cholecalciferol = 40 IU.

sunlight, whose dietary vitamin D intake is low (no dairy or lactose intolerant), or who wear head coverings (Gardiner et al. 2008).

The current dietary recommended intake for vitamin D for both pregnant and nonpregnant women is 15 µg per day in the form of cholecalciferol.

Calcium

Calcium is essential for bone development and maintenance throughout life and in pregnancy, and is important for the mineralization of fetal skeletal tissue. Many women in the United States do not consume the recommended amount of calcium during pregnancy and the growing fetus receives its total calcium supply from maternal sources. Therefore, if adequate bone has not been built before pregnancy and the maternal diet contains insufficient amounts, bone can be degraded as calcium is taken from the mother's skeleton (Table 1.5).

The Institute of Medicine (IOM) currently recommends 1,000 mg per day of calcium for both pregnant and nonpregnant women who are 19 to 50 years old, because the mineral is more efficiently absorbed during pregnancy. The recommendation is 1,300 mg per day for pregnant women who are younger than 19 years old.

Table 1.5 Selected food sources of calcium

Food	mg per serving	Percent DV*
Yogurt, plain, low fat, 8 oz	415	42
Mozzarella, part skim, 1.5 oz	333	33
Sardines, canned in oil, with bones, 3 oz	325	33
Yogurt, fruit, low fat, 8 oz	313–384	31–38
Cheddar cheese, 1.5 oz	307	31
Milk, nonfat, 8 oz	299	30
Soymilk, calcium-fortified, 8 oz	299	30
Milk, reduced-fat (2% milk fat), 8 oz	293	29
Milk, buttermilk, low fat, 8 oz	284	28
Milk, whole (3.25% milk fat), 8 oz	276	28
Orange juice, calcium-fortified, 6 oz	261	26
Tofu, firm, made with calcium sulfate, ½ cup	253	25
Salmon, pink, canned, solids with bone, 3 oz	181	18
Cottage cheese, 1% milk fat, 1 cup	138	14
Tofu, soft, made with calcium sulfate, ½ cup	138	14
Ready-to-eat cereal, calcium-fortified, 1 cup	100–1,000	10–100
Frozen yogurt, vanilla, soft serve, ½ cup	103	10
Turnip greens, fresh, boiled, ½ cup	99	10
Kale, raw, chopped, 1 cup	100	10
Kale, fresh, cooked, 1 cup	94	9
Ice cream, vanilla, ½ cup	84	8

Chinese cabbage, bok choi, raw, shredded, 1 cup	74	7
Bread, white, 1 slice	73	7
Pudding, chocolate, ready to eat, refrigerated, 4 oz	55	6
Tortilla, corn, ready-to-bake/fry, one 6 in. diameter	46	5
Tortilla, flour, ready-to-bake/fry, one 6 in. diameter	32	3
Sour cream, reduced fat, cultured, 2 tablespoons	31	3
Bread, whole-wheat, 1 slice	30	3
Broccoli, raw, ½ cup	21	2
Cheese, cream, regular, 1 tablespoon	14	1

Source: National Institutes of Health Office of Dietary Supplements (2013).
* DV = Daily Value. DVs were developed by the U.S. Food and Drug Administration to help consumers compare the nutrient contents among products within the context of a total daily diet.

Iodine

Iodine deficiency is one of the most preventable causes of brain damage throughout the world. Iodine is necessary for the production of thyroid hormones and must be acquired from the diet. Insufficient iodine intake leads to inadequate thyroid hormone production and iodine deficiency disorder, including abortion, stillbirth, mental retardation, **cretinism**, increased neonatal and infant mortality, goiter, and **hypothyroidism**. Iodine is readily transferred to the fetus whose thyroid concentrates the iodine and starts producing thyroid hormones by 10 to 12 weeks in utero. Therefore, adequate iodine intake is critical in the first half of pregnancy. In the United States, iodized salt is the primary source of iodine, followed by seafood. The recommendation for daily iodine intake is 150 µg for nonpregnant adults and 220 µg for pregnant women (Table 1.6).

Iron

Iron deficiency is the most common nutritional deficiency worldwide and the most common cause of anemia in pregnancy. Women of child-bearing age are at risk of iron deficiency because of blood loss from

Table 1.6 Selected food sources of iodine

Food	Approximate μg per serving	Percent DV* (%)
Seaweed, whole or sheet, 1 g	16–2,984	11–1,989
Cod, baked, 3 oz	99	66
Yogurt, plain, low-fat, 1 cup	75	50
Iodized salt, 1.5 g (approx. 1/4 teaspoon)	71	47
Milk, reduced fat, 1 cup	56	37
Fish sticks, 3 oz	54	36
Bread, white, enriched, 2 slices	45	30
Fruit cocktail in heavy syrup, canned, 1/2 cup	42	28
Shrimp, 3 oz	35	23
Ice cream, chocolate, 1/2 cup	30	20
Macaroni, enriched, boiled, 1 cup	27	18
Egg, 1 large	24	16
Tuna, canned in oil, drained, 3 oz	17	11
Corn, cream style, canned, 1/2 cup	14	9
Prunes, dried, 5 prunes	13	9
Cheese, cheddar, 1 oz	12	8
Raisin bran cereal, 1 cup	11	7
Lima beans, mature, boiled, 1/2 cup	8	5
Apple juice, 1 cup	7	5
Green peas, frozen, boiled, 1/2 cup	3	2
Banana, 1 medium	3	2

Source: National Institutes of Health Office of Dietary Supplements (2011).
* DV = Daily Value. DVs were developed by the U.S. Food and Drug Administration to help consumers compare the nutrient contents among products within the context of a total daily diet.

menstruation, poor diet, and frequent pregnancies. Iron needs are high during pregnancy and maternal reserves supply it to the developing placenta and fetal liver. Good food sources include meat, legumes, dried fruit, green leafy vegetables, eggs, and enriched bread and cereals. Iron deficiency anemia may lead to preterm birth and **intrauterine growth**

restriction. Recommendations for daily intake are 18 mg per day for nonpregnant women and 27 mg per day for pregnancy (Table 1.7).

Table 1.7 Selected food sources of iron

Food	mg per serving	Percent DV*
Breakfast cereals, fortified with 100% of the DV for iron, 1 serving	18	100
Oysters, eastern, cooked with moist heat, 3 oz	8	44
White beans, canned, 1 cup	8	44
Chocolate, dark, 45%–69% cacao solids, 3 oz	7	39
Beef liver, pan fried, 3 oz	5	28
Lentils, boiled and drained, ½ cup	3	17
Spinach, boiled and drained, ½ cup	3	17
Tofu, firm, ½ cup	3	17
Kidney beans, canned, ½ cup	2	11
Sardines, Atlantic, canned in oil, drained solids with bone, 3 oz	2	11
Chickpeas, boiled and drained, ½ cup	2	11
Tomatoes, canned, stewed, ½ cup	2	11
Beef, braised bottom round, trimmed to 1/8" fat, 3 oz	2	11
Potato, baked, flesh and skin, 1 medium potato	2	11
Cashew nuts, oil roasted, 1 oz (18 nuts)	2	11
Green peas, boiled, ½ cup	1	6
Chicken, roasted, meat and skin, 3 oz	1	6
Rice, white, long grain, enriched, parboiled, drained, ½ cup	1	6
Bread, whole wheat, 1 slice	1	6
Bread, white, 1 slice	1	6
Raisins, seedless, ¼ cup	1	6
Spaghetti, whole wheat, cooked, 1 cup	1	6
Tuna, bluefin, fresh, cooked with dry heat, 3 oz	1	6
Turkey, roasted, breast meat and skin, 3 oz	1	6
Nuts, pistachio, dry roasted, 1 oz (49 nuts)	1	6
Broccoli, boiled and drained, ½ cup	1	6

(*Continued*)

Table 1.7 Selected food sources of iron   (Continued)

Food	mg per serving	Percent DV*
Egg, hard boiled, 1 large	1	6
Rice, brown, long or medium grain, cooked, 1 cup	1	6
Cheese, cheddar, 1.5 oz	0	0
Cantaloupe, diced, ½ cup	0	0
Mushrooms, white, sliced and stir-fried, ½ cup	0	0
Cheese, cottage, 2% milk fat, ½ cup	0	0
Milk, 1 cup	0	0

Source: National Institutes of Health Office of Dietary Supplements (2015).
* DV = Daily Value. DVs were developed by the U.S. Food and Drug Administration to help consumers compare the nutrient contents among products within the context of a total daily diet.

Essential Fatty Acids

The **essential fatty acids** (EFA) linoleic acid (commonly known as omega-6s and found in vegetable oils) and alpha-linolenic acid (ALA) (commonly known as omega-3s and found in walnuts, flaxseeds, and canola oil) are important structural components of cell membranes, the central nervous system, and health of the cells in the retina of the eyes. EFAs cannot be synthesized in the body and must be ingested through food. The body can convert ALA into eicosapentaenoic acid (EPA) and docosahexaenonic acid (DHA), which are forms of omega-3s found abundantly in fatty fish, and are particularly important for fetal eye and brain development (Gardiner et al. 2008).

Because of high mercury levels detected in fish, the Food and Drug Administration (FDA) and the Environmental Protection Agency (EPA) issued an advisory in 2004 recommending that young children, pregnant women, nursing women, and women of childbearing age avoid consuming swordfish, king mackerel, shark, and tilefish. The warnings also recommended that those groups eat no more than 12 oz of fish and no more than 6 oz of canned albacore tuna per week (Food and Drug Administration 2014).

More recently, however, in order to encourage increased fish consumption among Americans due to the known health benefits of seafood, the FDA and EPA issued a draft advisory in June 2014 recommending

consumption of 8 to 12 oz of a variety of fish each week from choices that
are lower in mercury, such as salmon, shrimp, pollock, light canned tuna,
tilapia, catfish, and cod (Food and Drug Administration 2014).

Several studies have shown an association between maternal dietary
intake of fatty fish or oils providing EPA and DHA during pregnancy and
visual and cognitive development as well as motor activity in infants. However, there is mixed evidence for the effectiveness of these EFAs in preventing negative pregnancy outcomes during preconception and pregnancy. In
a review, the results of several randomized clinical studies have indicated
that supplementation with fish oils may lead to modest increases in gestation length, birth weight, or both (Gardiner et al. 2008) (Table 1.8).

There are several recommendations and guidelines addressing EFA
consumption for women. The IOM set the adequate intake (AI) for linoleic acid at 13 g per day for pregnant women and 12 g per day for women
18 to 50 years old. The AI for linolenic acid is 1.4 g per day for pregnant
women and 1.1 g per day for women 18 to 50 years old (Table 1.9).

*Table 1.8 Amounts of EPA and DHA in fish and fish oils, and the
amount of fish consumption required to provide about 1 g of EPA and
DHA per day*

	EPA + DHA content, g/3-oz serving fish (edible portion) or g/g oil	Amount required to provide ≈1 g of EPA + DHA per day, oz (fish) or g (oil)
Fish		
Tuna		
Light, canned in water, drained	0.26	12
White, canned in water, drained	0.73	4
Fresh	0.24–1.28	2.5–12
Sardines	0.98–1.70	2–3
Salmon		
Chum	0.68	4.5
Sockeye	0.68	4.5
Pink	1.09	2.5
Chinook	1.48	2

(Continued)

Table 1.8 Amounts of EPA and DHA in fish and fish oils, and the amount of fish consumption required to provide about 1 g of EPA and DHA per day   (Continued)

	EPA + DHA content, g/3-oz serving fish (edible portion) or g/g oil	Amount required to provide ≈1 g of EPA+DHA per day, oz (fish) or g (oil)
Atlantic, farmed	1.09–1.83	1.5–2.5
Atlantic, wild	0.9–1.56	2–3.5
Mackerel	0.34–1.57	2–8.5
Herring		
Pacific	1.81	1.5
Atlantic	1.71	2
Trout, rainbow		
Farmed	0.98	3
Wild	0.84	3.5
Halibut	0.4–1.0	3–7.5
Cod		
Pacific	0.13	23
Atlantic	0.24	12.5
Haddock	0.2	15
Catfish		
Farmed	0.15	20
Wild	0.2	15
Flounder/Sole	0.42	7
Oyster		
Pacific	1.17	2.5
Eastern	0.47	6.5
Farmed	0.37	8
Lobster	0.07–0.41	7.5–42.5
Crab, Alaskan King	0.35	8.5
Shrimp, mixed species	0.27	11
Clam	0.24	12.5
Scallop	0.17	17.5
Capsules		
Cod liver oil	0.19	5
Standard fish body oil	0.30	3
Omega-3 fatty acid concentrate	0.50	2

Data from the USDA Nutrient Data Laboratory. The intakes of fish given above are very rough estimates because oil content can vary markedly with species, season, diet, packaging, and cooking methods.
DHA: docosahexaenonic acid; EFA, essential fatty acids.

Source: Kris-Etherton, Harris, and Appel (2002).

Table 1.9 Alpha-linolenic acid content of selected vegetable oils, nuts, and seeds

	α-Linolenic acid content, g/tbsp
Olive oil	0.1
Walnuts, English	0.7
Soybean oil	0.9
Canola oil	1.3
Walnut oil	1.4
Flaxseeds	2.2
Flaxseed (linseed) oil	8.5

Source: Kris-Etherton, Harris, and Appel (2002).

Paternal Health

There are several reasons why preconception care for men is also important and improving men's preconception health can result in improved pregnancy outcomes. There are numerous ways that the DNA in sperm can be damaged, such as from exposure to tobacco, alcohol, drugs, caffeine, poor diet, radiation, chemotherapy, and testicular hyperthermia. Medical conditions such as diabetes mellitus, **varicoceles**, and **epididymitis**, if not treated, can also reduce sperm count and quality. However, since new sperm is created every 42 to 76 days, those that are damaged can be replaced. Therefore, male preconception care can offer an opportunity to improve sperm quality.

Weight and Nutrition for Men

Overweight and obesity among men is associated with lower testosterone level, poorer sperm quality, and reduced fertility, compared to nonoverweight or obese men; the chances of infertility increases by 10 percent for every 20 pounds a man is overweight. Therefore, an important medical care objective is to achieve a healthy weight before conception. It may be helpful for men to set weight loss goals for themselves, and work with a nutritionist or participate in a structured weight loss program (Frey et al. 2008).

A preconception nutritional screening should review current dietary patterns and use of restrictive diets, and evaluate nutrient intake. Nutrients of particular concern include levels of zinc and folate—they have antioxidant properties that protect sperm against oxidative stress and DNA damage. In a randomized controlled trial of 99 fertile and 94 subfertile men, daily administration of 66 mg of zinc sulfate and 5 mg of folic acid significantly increased sperm concentration of the subfertile men (Frey et al. 2008).

Other antioxidants have also been used to treat male infertility, including vitamin C, vitamin E, selenium, glutathione, ubiquinol, carnitine, and carotenoids. However, the safety and efficacy of such treatments have not been clearly established. In one study, the combination of vitamins C and E at high doses resulted in sperm DNA damage **in vitro**, raising concerns about the potential harms of high-dose antioxidant supplementation (Frey et al. 2008).

The CDC Prevention Checklist

As the benefits of preconception health gains increasing prominence in the scientific literature, the rise in attention to the issue has spurred public health promotion efforts to spread awareness. In 2013, the CDC launched a campaign called "Show the Love" designed to improve the health of women and babies by promoting preconception health and health care. The campaign's main goal is to increase the number of women who plan their pregnancies and engage in healthy behaviors before becoming pregnant. The campaign also focuses on steps that both women and men can take to reduce risks, promote healthy lifestyles, and increase readiness for pregnancy.

"Show Your Love" highlights the following interventions:

- Managing medical conditions (such as diabetes, obesity, phenylketonuria, sexually transmitted infections, hypothyroidism, seizure disorders, and HIV).

- Counseling women to avoid certain risks (such as alcohol consumption, smoking, prescription and over-the-counter teratogenic drug use, excess vitamin intake, undernutrition, and exposure to toxic substances).
- Counseling women to engage in healthy behaviors (such as reproductive life planning, folic acid consumption, and proper nutrition).
- Counseling women about the availability of vaccines to protect their infants from the consequences of infections that affect the mother (such as rubella, varicella, and hepatitis B).
- Counseling men to avoid certain risks (such as tobacco use and exposure to toxic substances).
- Counseling men to engage in healthy behaviors (such as reproductive life planning, proper nutrition, and healthy weight maintenance).

Source: Centers for Disease Control and Prevention (2015).

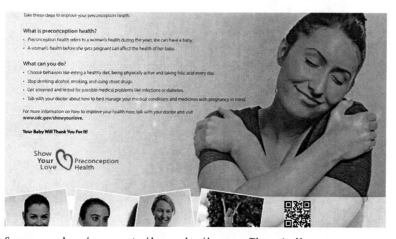

Source: www.cdc.gov/preconception/showyourlove/documents/Planner1.pdf

Key Terms

Amenorrhea
An abnormal absence of menstruation.

Beta-carotene
A red–orange pigment found in plants and fruits that can be converted by the body to vitamin A.

Body Mass Index
An index for assessing overweight and underweight obtained by dividing body weight in kilograms by height in meters squared. An index of 18.5 to 24.9 is considered normal BMI.

Bone Mineralization
The process of laying down minerals, such as calcium and phosphorous, within the fibrous matrix of the bone.

Carotenoids
Any of a class of mainly yellow, orange, or red fat-soluble pigments that give color to plant parts, such as carrots, tomatoes, and apricots.

Cesarean Delivery
The delivery of a baby through a surgical incision in the mother's abdomen and uterus.

Conception
The fertilization of an ovum by a sperm in the fallopian tube, followed by implantation in the uterus.

Congenital
Related to a disease or physical abnormality present from birth, whether inherited or caused by the environment, especially the uterine environment.

Cretinism
A condition of severely stunted physical and mental growth caused by a deficiency of thyroid hormone during fetal development.

Embryo
The human product of conception from implantation up to approximately the end of the second month of pregnancy.

Epididymitis
Inflammation of the tube at the back of the testicle that stores and carries sperm.

Epithelial
Related to the membranous tissue composed of one or more layers of cells that form the covering of most of the body's internal surfaces, such as the lining of vessels and cavities; and external surfaces, such as the skin.

Essential Fatty Acids
Fatty Acids that cannot be synthesized by the body and therefore must be obtained from food for normal physiologic function.

Fetus
Unborn offspring from the end of the eighth week after conception to the moment of birth.

Gene Expression
The process by which genetic instructions are used to make gene products—usually protein molecules—that go on to perform essential functions, such as enzymes, hormones, and receptors.

Genetic Reprogramming
Refers to environmentally influenced epigenetic changes or "marks" on DNA that either activate or suppress certain genes, thereby "reprogramming" cells to behave in a certain way.

Gestation
The period of fetal development from conception until birth; about 266 days in humans.

Gestational Diabetes
Diabetes that occurs during pregnancy, and typically resolves after birth.

Glycated Hemoglobin
A protein contained inside red blood cells that binds with glucose in the blood, therefore becoming "glycated." A measurement of glycated hemoglobin offers an indication of average blood sugar levels over a period of weeks or months.

Hypothyroidism
An abnormality of the thyroid gland characterized by insufficient production of thyroid hormone, which can result in a decreased basal metabolic rate, causing weight gain and fatigue.

Implantation
The process by which a fertilized egg in the blastocyst stage of development implants in the uterine lining.

In vitro
Performed or taking place in a test tube, culture dish, or elsewhere outside a living organism.

Infertility
A condition in which a couple has problems conceiving, or getting pregnant, after one year of regular sexual intercourse without using any birth control methods.

Intrauterine Growth Restriction
A condition in which a baby doesn't grow to normal weight during pregnancy.

Macrosomia
A newborn that is significantly larger than average.

Neonatal
Of or relating to newborn children, especially in the first week of life and up to four weeks old.

Neural Tube Defect
Any of a group of congenital abnormalities involving the brain and spinal cord, including spina bifida, caused by the failure of the neural tube to close properly during embryonic development.

Osteoporosis
A medical condition in which the bones become increasingly porous, brittle, and vulnerable to fractures due to the depletion of calcium and protein in the skeletal system.

Periconceptional
The period from before conception to early pregnancy.

Preconception
The time prior to pregnancy.

Placenta

The vascular organ formed in the uterus during pregnancy, consisting of both maternal and embryonic tissues, and providing oxygen and nutrients for the fetus and transfer of waste products from the fetal to the maternal blood circulation.

Preeclampsia

A syndrome occurring in a pregnant woman after her 20th week of pregnancy that causes high blood pressure, excess protein in the urine, swelling in the face and hands, and headache.

Preterm Birth

Also called premature birth; birth that occurs before the 37th week of pregnancy.

Retinoids

A class of chemical compounds that are related to vitamin A and function like it in the body.

Small-for-Gestational-Age

Infants who are smaller in size than normal with a birth weight below the 10th percentile for gestational age.

Stillbirth

The birth of a dead infant.

Teratogenic

The ability of a drug or other substance to interfere with the development of a fetus, causing birth defects.

Varicocele

An abnormal enlargement of the veins within the scrotum.

References

Centers for Disease Control and Prevention. n.d. "Action Plan for the National Initiative on Preconception Health and Health Care (PCHHC): Introduction." www.cdc.gov/preconception/documents/ActionPlanNationalInitiativePCHHC2012-2014.pdf (accessed June 23, 2015).

Centers for Disease Control and Prevention. July 31, 2015. "Preconception Health and Health Care." www.cdc.gov/preconception/hcp/index.html (accessed August 4, 2015).

Dean, S.V., Z.S. Lassi, A.M. Imam, and Z.A. Bhutta. September 2014. "Preconception Care: Nutritional Risks and Interventions." *Reproductive Health* 11, Suppl. 3, p. S3.

Dunlop, A.L., B.W. Jack, J.N. Bottalico, M.C. Lu, A. James, C.S. Shellhaas, L.H. Hallstrom, B.D. Solomon, W.G. Feero, M.K. Menard, and M.R. Prasad. December 2008. "The Clinical Content of Preconception Care: Women with Chronic Medical Conditions." *American Journal of Obstetrics and Gynecology* 199, no. 6, Suppl. 2, pp. 310–27.

Food and Drug Administration. June 10, 2014. "New Advice: Pregnant Women and Young Children Should Eat More Fish." www.fda.gov/ForConsumers/ConsumerUpdates/ucm397443.htm (accessed August 10, 2015).

Frey, K.A., S.M. Navarro, M. Kotelchuck, and M.C. Lu. December 2008. "The Clinical Content of Preconception Care: Preconception Care for Men." *Journal of Obstetrics and Gynecology* 199, no. 6, Suppl. 2, pp. 389–95.

Gardiner, P.M., L. Nelson, C.S. Shellhaas, A.L. Dunlop, R. Long, S. Andrist, and B.W. Jack. December 2008. "The Clinical Content of Preconception Care: Nutrition and Dietary Supplements." *American Journal of Obstetrics and Gynecology* 199, no. 6, Suppl. 2, pp. 345–56.

Healthy People 2020. n.d. "Maternal, Infant, and Child Objectives." www.healthypeople.gov/2020/topics-objectives/topic/maternal-infant-and-child-health/objectives (accessed July 4, 2015).

Kris-Etherton, P.M., W.S. Harris, and L.J. Appel. November 2002. "Fish Consumption, Fish Oil, Omega-3 Fatty Acids, and Cardiovascular Disease." *Circulation* 106, no. 21, pp. 2747–57.

Lassi, Z.S., A.M. Imam, S.V. Dean, and Z.A. Bhutta. September 2014. "Preconception Care: Screening and Management of Chronic Disease and Promoting Psychological Health." *Reproductive Health* 11, Suppl. 3, p. S5.

Linabery, A.M., R.W. Nahhas, W. Johnson, A.C. Choh, B. Towne, A.O. Odegaard, S.A. Czerwinski, and E.W. Demerath. 2014. "Stronger Influence of Maternal Than Paternal Obesity on Infant and Early Childhood Body Mass Index: The Fels Longitudinal Study." *Reproductive Health* 11, Suppl. 3, p. S3.

Mumford, S.L., K.A. Michels, N. Salaria, P. Valanzasca, and J.M. Belizán. October 2014. "Preconception Care: It's Never Too Eary." *Reproductive Health* 11, no. 1, p. 73.

National Conference of State Legislatures. May 2011. "Healthy People 2020 and Maternal and Child Health." www/ncsl.org/research/health/healthy-people-2020-and-maternal-and-child-health.aspx (accessed July 7, 2015).

National Institutes of Health Office of Dietary Supplements. June 24, 2011." Iodine Fact Sheet for Health Professionals." https://ods.od.nih.gov/factsheets/Iodine-HealthProfessional/#h3 (accessed July 8, 2015).

National Institutes of Health Office of Dietary Supplements. December 14, 2012. "Folate Fact Sheet for Health Professionals." https://ods.od.nih.gov/pdf/factsheets/Folate-Consumer.pdf (accessed July 8, 2015).

National Institutes of Health Office of Dietary Supplements. November 21, 2013. "Calcium Fact Sheet for Health Professionals." https://ods.od.nih.gov/factsheets/Calcium-HealthProfessional/#h3 (accessed July 8, 2015).

National Institutes of Health Office of Dietary Supplements. June 5, 2013. "Vitamin A Fact Sheet for Health Professionals." https://ods.od.nih.gov/factsheets/VitaminA-HealthProfessional/#h3 (accessed July 8, 2015).

National Institutes of Health Office of Dietary Supplements. November 10, 2014. "Vitamin D Fact Sheet for Health Professionals." https://ods.od.nih.gov/factsheets/VitaminD-HealthProfessional/#3 (accessed July 8, 2015).

National Institutes of Health Office of Dietary Supplements. November 24, 2015. "Iron Fact Sheet for Health Professionals." https://ods.od.nih.gov/factsheets/Iron-HealthProfessional/#h3 (accessed December 1, 2015).

CHAPTER 2

Nutrition for a Healthy Pregnancy

Introduction

At no other time in the human life cycle are growth and development more rapid and dramatic than during pregnancy. A normal pregnancy lasts about 40 weeks (from the start of the last menstrual period to birth). An infant born before the 37th week of pregnancy is considered to be preterm. Pregnancy begins with a single fertilized egg that grows into a fully developed newborn weighing on an average 3,500 g. During this period of gestation (which is commonly divided into trimesters of about 13 weeks each), maternal nutrient needs significantly increase in order to support the demands of the fetus. If the mother's nutrient intake is inadequate to meet these demands, fetal growth and development are compromised. This chapter focuses on specific nutrient requirements for

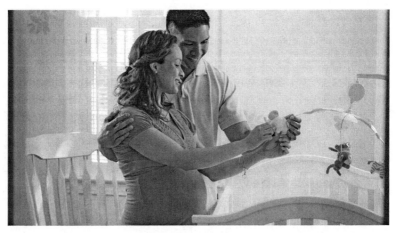

Source: https://wicworks.fns.usda.gov/nal_web/wicworks//resources/WICImages/Image35-300DPI.tif

a healthy pregnancy, as well as considerations related to specific complications, such as gestational diabetes and pregnancy-induced hypertension.

Fetal Development

The start of a new human life begins with one cell—the fertilized egg. As a woman's ovary prepares to release an ovum (female egg), it forms the *corpus luteum*, a tissue about 12 mm in diameter, within the follicle that releases the egg. This small mass of tissue produces two important hormones, **estrogen** and **progesterone**, which stimulate the development of the *endometrium* (the inner lining of the uterus). Fertilization takes place at the end of the **fallopian tube** and comes to fruition once the genetic material of a sperm combines with that of an ovum to form a fertilized egg known as a **zygote**.

Propelled by **peristalsis** and **cilia**, the zygote travels along the tube to the uterus while its cells divide rapidly through *mitosis*—forming two cells, then four cells, then eight cells and so on. These rapidly dividing cells eventually form a hollow ball known as a **blastocyst**, which implants itself in the uterine wall. In rare cases, the fertilized egg remains in the fallopian tube creating a *tubal pregnancy* or *ectopic pregnancy*, which is dangerous to the mother. The blastocyst secretes a hormone called **human chorionic gonadotropin** (hCG), which signals the corpus luteum to continue producing hormones.

Once the ovum is fertilized, it will embed itself in the uterine wall within 8 to 10 days. The dividing fertilized egg also produces hormones that signal the corpus luteum to continue its production of estrogen and progesterone.

By day 10 to 12, an amniotic sac begins to form, and at this point, the implanted blastocyst is considered to be an embryo. The amniotic sac fills with a clear liquid (amniotic fluid) and surrounds the developing embryo. While some of the blastocyst's cells form the embryo, other cells become the placenta.

It is important to note that health care providers date pregnancy from the first day of the woman's last menstrual period, which is typically two weeks before fertilization. By about three weeks after fertilization, which equals five weeks of pregnancy, most organs have begun to form, including the beating heart, spinal cord, and brain.

At eight weeks of pregnancy, the placenta forms tiny hair-like projections (villi) that extend into the wall of the uterus, and is fully formed by 18 to 20 weeks, but continues to grow throughout pregnancy. At delivery, the placenta weighs about one pound. A thin membrane separates the embryo's blood in the villi from the mother's blood that flows through the space surrounding the villi. Since the embryo's lungs and digestive system are not yet functioning, all nutrient, excretory, and gas exchanges occur through the placenta. Nutrients and oxygen move from the mother's blood into the embryo's blood, and waste materials move in the opposite direction. The placenta also prevents the woman's immune system from attacking the embryo because the maternal antibodies are too large to pass through the membrane.

At the end of the eighth week after fertilization (10 weeks of pregnancy), the embryo is considered a **fetus** and is more than half an inch

Table 2.1 *Stages of fetal development*

Stage of development	Weeks of pregnancy
Last menstrual period before fertilization	0
Fertilization. Zygote begins to develop into a hollow ball of cells known as a blastocyst.	2
The blastocyst implants in the uterine wall and the amniotic sac begins to form.	3
The brain and spinal cord (neural tube) begin to develop.	5
The heart and major blood vessels are developing. Heart beat can be detected.	6
The beginnings of arms and legs appear.	7
Bones and muscles form. The face and neck develop. Brain waves can be detected. The skeleton is formed. Defined fingers and toes.	9
The kidneys begin to function. Almost all organs are completely formed. The fetus can move.	10
The fetus' sex can be identified and it can hear.	14
The fetus' fingers can grasp, and it moves more vigorously, so that the mother can feel it. The fetus' body begins to fill out as fat is deposited beneath the skin. Hair appears on the head and skin; and eyebrows and eyelashes are present.	16

(Continued)

Table 2.1 Stages of fetal development   *(Continued)*

Stage of development	Weeks of pregnancy
The placenta is fully formed.	20
The fetus has a chance of survival outside the uterus.	24
The fetus is active, changing positions often, and its head moves into position for delivery.	25
Delivery	37–42

Source: Merck Manuals (n.d.).

long. In the months that follow, growth and organ specialization domi-
nate its development. At this point, the placenta produces enough progesterone, estrogen, and other hormones to help maintain the pregnancy,
so that the corpus luteum is no longer necessary and it becomes inactive.

By about 10 weeks after fertilization (which equals 12 weeks of pregnancy), almost all of the fetus' organs are formed, except its brain and
spinal cord, which continue to form and develop throughout pregnancy.
The first 10 weeks of pregnancy is the period when malformations (birth
defects) are most likely to occur, so the embryo is most vulnerable to the
impact of drugs, radiation, and viruses.

By the 12th week after fertilization (14 weeks of pregnancy), the
fetus' sex can be identified, and at 14 to 18 weeks after fertilization (16 to
20 weeks of pregnancy), the mother can feel the fetus moving. By about
22 weeks after fertilization (24 weeks of pregnancy), the fetus has a chance
of surviving outside the uterus. Table 2.1 summarizes some of the milestones in embryonic and fetal development.

The Placenta

The placenta is about a 9-in. long, 1-in. thick temporary organ that forms
in the uterus of the pregnant woman, connecting the developing fetus to
the uterine wall and allowing nutrient uptake, waste elimination, and gas
exchange by way of the mother's blood supply. There are two components
that comprise the placenta: the *fetal placenta*, which develops from the
same blastocyst that forms the fetus; and the *maternal placenta*, which
develops from uterine tissue. The development of the maternal blood

supply to the placenta is complete by the end of the first trimester of pregnancy, but the placenta itself continues to grow throughout pregnancy.

The fetus is connected to the placenta via an **umbilical cord** that is approximately 22 to 24 in. long. The umbilical cord is comprised of three blood vessels: one large umbilical vein and two smaller umbilical arteries. The umbilical vein carries blood containing nutrients and oxygen to the fetus. The umbilical arteries transport deoxygenated fetal blood, carbon dioxide, and other waste material from the fetus to the placenta. At the junction of the umbilical cord and placenta, the umbilical blood vessels branch out to form smaller and smaller blood vessels, bringing the fetal blood extremely close to the maternal blood. The fingerlike projections containing fetal blood vessels extend into the area of the mother's blood, but no intermingling of fetal and maternal blood occurs, and substances pass back and forth by **passive diffusion**, **facilitated diffusion**, **active transport**, and **endocytosis**.

The period from just after the child is born until the placenta is expelled from the mother's body is called the *third stage of labor*, which typically happens 15 to 30 minutes after birth.

In addition to being a source of oxygen and nutrients for the fetus, the placenta also secretes hormones that are important during pregnancy. If the mother's nutrient reserves are inadequate during placental development, no amount of nutrients later on in pregnancy can make up for the depletion. If the placenta fails to form or function properly, the fetus will not receive optimal nourishment.

The fetal part of the placenta releases hCG, which stimulates the corpus luteum of the ovary to continue producing estrogen and progesterone. By the third month of pregnancy, the placenta assumes the job of producing estrogen and progesterone itself, and the corpus luteum becomes inactive. The high estrogen and progesterone blood levels maintain the lining of the uterus and prepare the breasts for producing milk. Meanwhile, the placenta also releases **human placental lactogen** (hPL), which works in conjunction with estrogen and progesterone in preparing the breasts for **lactation**. **Relaxin** is another placental hormone that allows the mother's pelvic ligaments and cervix to relax and become more flexible in preparation for birth.

If the placenta fails to function properly, it can limit the nutrient supply to the fetus and hinder fetal growth. Intrauterine growth restriction leads to babies being born with depleted fat and glycogen stores. There is increasing evidence that maternal factors, including body mass index (BMI), gestational weight gain, physical activity level, and smoking, as well as diseases related to the placenta, can affect fetal growth and pregnancy outcomes (Brett et al. 2014).

Weight Gain During Pregnancy

Studies show that weight gain before pregnancy as well as during pregnancy can impact not only the immediate outcomes for the mother and the baby, but also their long-term health. The prevalence of obesity among pregnant women is on the rise and is associated with adverse maternal and newborn outcomes. Women who are obese before pregnancy are much more likely to develop gestational diabetes, preeclampsia, longer labors, and give birth by cesarean delivery. The risks to the fetus include: miscarriage, birth defects, macrosomia, **shoulder dystocia**, stillbirth, and **neonatal** death (Agha, Agha, and Sandell 2014).

Compared to normal-weight women, babies whose mothers were obese during pregnancy are also at a higher risk for developing type 2 diabetes, and for developing it at a younger age than those whose mothers were not obese during pregnancy (National Institute of Child Health and Human Development 2011).

The old cliché about pregnant women needing to "eat for two" has encouraged many mothers-to-be to consume far more calories than they need during pregnancy, leading to excessive weight gain. A pregnant woman only requires about 350 to 450 additional calories daily to adequately support fetal growth. The Institute of Medicine (IOM) recommends that all pregnant women should gain on average 1.1 to 4.4 pounds during the first trimester, and then follow the guidelines for total weight gain by the end of pregnancy as outlined in Table 2.2 based on pre-pregnancy BMI (Institute of Medicine 2015).

The American College of Obstetricians and Gynecologists (ACOG) recommends the following rate of weight gain during the second and third trimesters of pregnancy: 1 to 1.3 pounds per week if pre-pregnancy BMI is

Table 2.2 Recommended total weight gain for pregnancy*

Pre-pregnancy BMI	Recommended total weight gain
<18.5 kg/m² underweight	28–40 lb (12.5–18 kg)
18.5 to <24.9 kg/m² normal weight	25–35 lb (11.5–16 kg)
25–29.9 kg/m² overweight	15–25 lb (7–11.5 kg)
>30 kg/m² obese	11–20 lb (5–9 kg)

Source: Institute of Medicine of National Academy of Sciences (2009).

* For twins the provisional recommendations for weight gain during pregnancy issued by the Institute of Medicine are:
Normal weight women should gain 37–54 lb (17–25 kg)
Overweight women should gain 31–50 lb (14–23 kg)
Obese women should gain 25–42 lb (11–19 kg)

below 18.5 kg/m²; 0.8 to 1 pounds per week for pre-pregnancy BMIs in the normal range; 0.5 to 0.7 lbs per week if pre-pregnancy BMI is categorized as overweight; and 0.4 to 0.6 lbs per week for all pre-pregnancy BMI categories that indicate obesity (ACOG 2013). An insufficient or low maternal weight gain during the second or third trimester increases the risk for **intrauterine growth restriction**. Table 2.2 summarizes the recommended total weight gain for pregnancy.

It is important to keep in mind that these recommendations are guidelines. The calorie needs and total weight gain required for pregnancy varies among women depending on activity level, body composition, health status, and other factors. However, a sudden sharp increase in weight after the 20th week of pregnancy may indicate abnormal water retention and should be watched closely, especially if there is a rise in blood pressure, and protein is found in the mother's urine (proteinuria).

Weight Distribution

The extra weight normally gained by women during pregnancy is derived from a variety of sources including the baby itself, placenta, amniotic fluid, uterus, maternal blood, fluids in maternal tissue, and maternal fat and nutrient stores. The average weight of a newborn is about 7.5 pounds. During the third trimester, the mother acquires extra **adipose tissue**, which is necessary for maternal energy reserves to support the rapidly growing fetus and for maintaining lactation after birth. During pregnancy, the woman's heart must work harder to pump more blood to the

Table 2.3 Weight distribution during pregnancy

Weight (lb)	Purpose
7.5	Baby (average weight)
7	Extra stored protein, fat, and other nutrients
4	Blood
4	Other extra body fluids
2	Breast enlargement
2	Uterine enlargement
2	Amniotic fluid
1.5	The placenta

Source: The Nemours Foundation (2013).

uterus; and the amount of blood pumped by the heart (cardiac output) increases by 30 to 50 percent. The total volume of blood increases by almost 50 percent during pregnancy, which accounts for some of the weight gain. The amount of fluid in the blood increases, diluting the number of oxygen-carrying red blood cells, so blood tests often indicate mild anemia, which is normal. Table 2.3 summarizes the weight distribution that occurs during pregnancy; and Table 2.4 highlights the purpose, major food sources, and recommended amounts of key nutrients that are important for pregnancy.

Nutrient Requirements During Pregnancy

During pregnancy, the mother and her developing fetus undergo dramatic physiological changes that increase the woman's needs for most essential nutrients and also for energy. Studies show that a healthy and balanced diet during pregnancy improves infant outcomes, including reduction of fetal and infant mortality, intrauterine growth restriction, low birth weight, premature birth, and decreased incidence of birth defects (Nnam 2015).

Ideally, the expectant mother's nutrient intake should follow the guidelines specified by the IOM's Dietary Reference Intake (DRI), and meal patterns should correspond to the type and quantity of foods recommended in the *Choose My Plate* meal plans. More information can be obtained at www.choosemyplate.gov/moms-daily-food-plan.

Table 2.4 *Food sources of key nutrients and recommended dietary intake*

Nutrient	Purpose	Major food sources	DRI
Protein	Cell growth and blood production.	Lean meat, fish, poultry, eggs, beans, peanut butter, tofu.	71 g
Carbohydrates	Daily energy production.	Breads, cereals, rice, potatoes, pasta, fruits, vegetables, dairy products.	175 g
Fat	Body energy stores. Brain and eye development from essential fatty acids.	Meat, whole milk dairy products, nuts, peanut butter, butter, vegetable oils, fatty fish.	14 g Linoleic acid 1.6 g Linolenic acid
Calcium	Formation of fetal skeleton.	Milk, cheese, yogurt, sardines or salmon with bones, fortified orange juice.	1,000 mg
Iron	Hemoglobin production.	Lean red meat, spinach, iron-fortified whole-grain breads and cereals.	27 mg
Iodine	Synthesis of thyroid hormones, which regulate cell metabolism.	Iodized salt, seafood.	220 µg
Vitamin A	Healthy skin, good eyesight, growing bones.	Carrots, dark leafy greens, sweet potatoes.	770 µg RAE
Vitamin C	Healthy gums, teeth, and bones; enhances iron absorption.	Citrus fruit, broccoli, tomatoes, strawberries, kiwi.	85 mg

(Continued)

Table 2.4 Food sources of key nutrients and recommended dietary intake   (Continued)

Nutrient	Purpose	Major food sources	DRI
Vitamin B12	Formation of red blood cells, maintaining nervous system health.	Meat, fish, poultry, milk, supplements.	2.6 μg
Vitamin D	Healthy bones and teeth; aids absorption of calcium and phosphorus.	Fortified milk and other dairy products, fortified soymilk, egg yolks, fatty fish.	15 μg
Folate	Formation of red blood cells.	Green leafy vegetables, dark yellow fruits and vegetables, beans, peas, nuts.	600 μg
Choline	Formation of cell membrane; nervous system signaling.	Seafood, egg yolks, collard greens, broccoli, Swiss chard, asparagus.	450 mg

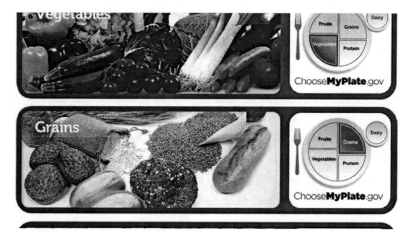

Source: www.choosemyplate.gov/printable-materials

Energy

Energy requirements during pregnancy increase mainly due to the synthesis of fat storage for both the mother and the fetus, and to spare protein reserves. The mother's cardiovascular, respiratory, and renal systems must work harder to support her higher basal metabolic needs, and therefore her daily calorie intake must be sufficient to fuel her body's added workload. The DRI standard recommends an additional amount of energy of approximately 340 kcal per day during the second trimester and 452 kcal per day during the third trimester of pregnancy. The total daily calorie intake during middle and late pregnancy should be based on the woman's nonpregnant estimated energy requirement plus the additional energy needed. Measured adequate weight gain during pregnancy is a reliable indication of whether enough calories are being consumed (Food and Nutrition Board, Institute of Medicine of the National Academies 2005).

Carbohydrate

As for nonpregnant adults, the IOM recommends that pregnant women consume approximately 45 to 65 percent of their total calorie intake from carbohydrates. At minimum, they should get 175 g of carbohydrates per day (Institute of Medicine 2005) to meet the fetal brain's need for glucose.

Foods such as vegetables, fruits, and whole-grain bread and cereal products that contain fiber are good high-carbohydrate choices.

Protein

Pregnant women require additional protein to support rapid fetal growth, as well as the growth of the uterus, mammary glands, and placenta. Additional protein is also required for the formation of amniotic fluid and to create reserves for labor, delivery, and lactation. The total amount of protein recommended for a pregnant woman is 71 g per day, an increase of 25 g (Institute of Medicine 2005). Milk, eggs, cheese, and meat are good choices for complete protein foods as they contain all nine essential amino acids. Additional protein may be obtained from legumes and whole grains. Vegetarian diets are adequate to meet protein needs for pregnancy provided that the woman consumes a variety of plant-based complementary protein sources.

Fat

Dietary fat provides an energy source for fetal growth and development and is important for proper absorption of fat-soluble vitamins. The adequate macronutrient distribution range recommended by the IOM is 20 to 35 percent of total calories. As explained in Chapter 1, certain fats also provide essential fatty acids known as alpha-linolenic (omega-3 fatty acids) and linoleic acid (omega-6 fatty acids). They are considered to be long chain polyunsaturated fatty acids that contribute to the structural components of cell membranes and are particularly important for the fetus' visual and cognitive development (Krauss-Etschmann et al. 2007). Rich food sources of linoleic acid include safflower, corn, sunflower, and soy oil. Alpha-linolenic acid is found in flaxseed, walnut, soybean and canola oils, and leafy green vegetables. The DRI for these essential fatty acids is 10 percent of total calories.

Two important subtypes of alpha-linolenic fatty acids are eicosapentaenoic acid (EPA) and docosahexaenoic acid (DHA), which play particularly important roles in pregnancy. EPA and DHA can be derived from food sources of alpha-linolenic acid, but only in small amounts. So, adequate intake (AI) of these two omega-3 fatty acids depends on the consumption of their direct food sources or the use of supplements. Fish and seafood are by far the richest sources of EPA and DHA (see Table 1.8 in Chapter 1 for EPA and DHA content of select food sources).

The Food and Drug Administration (FDA) recommends that pregnant women consume at least 8 to 12 oz of a variety of fish and seafood per week, with no more than 6 oz of white (albacore) tuna (Food and Drug Administration 2014). Many pregnant women avoid eating fish during pregnancy because they are fearful of the mercury content of these foods. The FDA, therefore, encourages women to select different types of fish and seafood that are known to be low in mercury, such as shrimp, canned light tuna, salmon, pollock, and catfish. Fish that are known to contain high levels of mercury include swordfish, king mackerel, tilefish, and shark, and should not be consumed during pregnancy.

Vitamins and Minerals

Folate

Folate is a term that refers to multiple forms of this essential water-soluble B-complex vitamin, which plays a role in the formation of red blood cells. It naturally occurs in plant foods, while *folic acid* is a synthetic form that is used in fortified foods and dietary supplements. Folic acid is significantly more bioavailable than folate, and AI reduces the occurrence of neural tube defects (Bailey, West, and Black 2015). Folate plays an important role in the production of red blood cells and helps the neural tube develop into the brain and spinal cord. All women, including adolescents, who are capable of becoming pregnant, should consume 400 μg per day of folic acid from fortified foods, as well as foods naturally rich in folate. Pregnant women are advised to consume 600 μg of folate or folic acid equivalents per day.

Vitamin A

Vitamin A is a fat-soluble vitamin that is important for cell differentiation, reproduction, and organ and bone formation. Too little intake of vitamin A can impair fetal growth. However, an excessively high intake in its pure form of retinol or retinoic acid through use of supplements or topical creams can result in severe birth defects. Foods such as carrots, sweet potatoes, and cantaloupe that are rich in beta-carotene, a precursor to vitamin A, do not pose a risk for vitamin A toxicity. The tolerable upper intake level (UL) for pregnancy is 3,000 µg retinol activity equivalents (RAE) per day. The DRI is 770 µg RAE per day.

Vitamin D

Because of the fetus' high need for the minerals calcium and phosphorous to form its skeletal tissue, vitamin D is needed to promote the absorption and use of these nutrients. The daily recommended amount for pregnancy is 15 µg of cholecalciferol (600 IU per day), which is the same as for nonpregnant women. Food sources include fortified milk, fortified fruit juices, egg yolks, and fortified margarine. Women who have adequate exposure to sunlight likely do not need much more additional vitamin D.

Choline

Choline is an essential nutrient for the normal function of all cells as well as **stem cell** proliferation. Maternal deficiency can interfere with normal fetal brain development (Zeisel 2006). The majority of pregnant women are not achieving the AI for pregnancy of 450 mg of choline per day (Procter and Campbell 2014).

Iron

Iron is a mineral that is an essential component of hemoglobin synthesis and is critical for optimal growth and **cognitive** function. Iron deficiency is the most common micronutrient deficiency worldwide, and is especially common during pregnancy because of the extra blood acquired by the mother and the demands made by fetal growth and development. Adequate iron is also necessary to allow the newborn to store enough for the first few months of life. Maternal iron deficiency is associated with low birth weight and premature delivery; and children who are born to iron-deficient mothers are more likely to have low iron reserves, suffer from impaired physical and cognitive development, and to have weaker immune function (Bailey, West, and Black 2015).

The IOM recommends that all pregnant women consume 27 mg of iron per day, a 50 percent increase compared with the daily recommendation for nonpregnant women.

Calcium

During pregnancy, calcium is necessary for the mineralization of the fetus' skeleton, and for the maintenance of maternal bone health. Since calcium absorption from food increases and urinary excretion of the mineral decreases, the DRI for calcium, which is 1,000 mg per day, is the same for pregnant women as it is for nonpregnant women of childbearing age.

Iodine

Iodine is a trace mineral required for normal brain development and growth. Maternal requirements increase during pregnancy. National surveys find that some pregnant and lactating women have an inadequate dietary intake of iodine (Procter and Campbell 2014). The IOM recommends a daily intake of 220 μg per day for pregnancy.

Gestational Hypertension and Preeclampsia

Chronic high blood pressure, also known as hypertension, occurs when arteries carrying blood from the heart to the body's organs are narrowed, causing pressure to increase in these blood vessels. During pregnancy, gestational hypertension may develop after week 20 and can make it difficult for blood to reach the placenta. Such reduced blood flow can hinder the growth of the fetus and place the mother at higher risk of preterm labor and a more serious form of high blood pressure known as preeclampsia.

Preeclampsia is a serious medical condition characterized by chronic hypertension and protein in the urine. It can lead to *eclampsia*, which involves the development of seizures or coma. Hypertensive disorders including gestational hypertension and preeclampsia affect up to

10 percent of pregnant women (Austdal et al. 2015); and treatment is usually the early delivery of the baby through a cesarean section. Some risk factors for preeclampsia include:

- Preeclampsia in a previous pregnancy
- Existing conditions such as high blood pressure, diabetes, and kidney disease
- Being 35 years of age or older; or younger than age 20
- Carrying two or more fetuses
- Obesity
- Being African American.

Gestational Diabetes

Gestational diabetes occurs when a woman who did not have diabetes prior to her pregnancy develops the condition during pregnancy. Diabetes is the failure of the body to utilize the hormone insulin sufficiently enough to keep blood sugar levels within a normal range. In gestational diabetes, the hormonal changes involved in pregnancy cause the pancreas to either not make enough **insulin**, or causes the body not to use it normally. Instead, the glucose builds up in the blood.

The prevalence of gestational diabetes in the United States is 9.2 percent of pregnant women (American Diabetes Association 2014) and is more common among obese adults, women with a family history of diabetes, and certain ethnic groups, such Native Americans, Pacific Islanders, and those of Mexican, Indian, or Asian descent.

When uncontrolled, gestational diabetes can increase the risk of health problems for pregnant women and the possibility of fetal death. Poor diabetic control also increases the risk of miscarriage and birth defects. Babies born to women with diabetes tend to be larger than those born to women without diabetes, and these newborns may be particularly large, creating complications during delivery (Friel 2015).

To reduce the chances of complications during pregnancy, blood sugar levels should be maintained as close to normal as possible. Pregnant women who have diabetes are advised to follow an appropriate diet to stabilize blood sugar, usually by monitoring the amount and type of carbohydrates eaten; balancing choices from all food groups; and consuming reasonable portion sizes. Treatment may also include regular exercise, and possibly use of an oral hypoglycemic agent (drug that lowers blood sugar), or exogenous insulin.

After delivery, gestational diabetes usually disappears. However, many women who have gestational diabetes are at higher risk of developing type 2 diabetes later in their lives.

Iron-Deficiency Anemia

Because of the amount of blood they produce throughout pregnancy, expectant mothers need additional iron (see previous section on iron in this chapter). Iron-deficiency anemia is fairly common and is prevalent among 16.2 percent of all pregnant women in the United States (U.S. Preventative Services Task Force 2015). The symptoms of an iron deficiency include fatigue, shortness of breath, and pale skin. The IOM recommends 27 mg of iron daily to reduce the risk for iron-deficiency anemia.

Hyperemesis Gravidarum

Nausea and vomiting are common in the first few weeks of pregnancy and sometimes throughout the entire length of gestation. However, hyperemesis gravidarum is severe and persistent nausea and vomiting that may result in weight loss, nutritional deficiencies, as well as abnormal electrolyte balance and dehydration. The condition occurs in 0.5 to 2 percent of all pregnancies; peaks at 8 to 12 weeks of pregnancy, and typically resolves by week 20. The cause of hyperemesis gravidarum is not known, and it often requires treatment with IV fluids, sometimes hospitalization for several days, and use of **antiemetics** (Wilcox 2013).

Constipation and Heartburn

Between 11 and 38 percent of women experience constipation during pregnancy, which is likely caused by rising progesterone levels and is typically managed through increasing fiber and fluid intake, as well as using bulk-forming laxatives if necessary (Vazquez 2010).

Heartburn is one of the most common gastrointestinal symptoms experienced by pregnant women with a prevalence of about 22 percent in the first trimester, going up to between 62 and 72 percent in the third trimester. During pregnancy, the lower esophageal sphincter gets displaced in the chest cavity allowing food and acidic contents to pass from the stomach into the esophagus, causing a "burning" sensation. Pressure from the growing uterus worsens the condition. Most cases can be managed with dietary changes and lifestyle modifications, such as small frequent meals, remaining in an upright position soon after eating, and wearing loose clothing. If there's no relief, then calcium-based antacids can be used (Vazquez 2010).

Prenatal Supplements

Generally, most of a pregnant woman's nutrient needs can be obtained from a well-planned and balanced diet. However, certain nutrients such as iron and vitamin D (if there is inadequate sun exposure) may be challenging to consume in sufficient amounts. Most doctors recommend a prenatal supplement, but they should not be relied upon to make up for an unhealthy diet. Foods provide antioxidants, fiber, and other substances that are not found in dietary supplements. Supplementary forms of vitamins and minerals may benefit women who routinely do not maintain an adequate diet; have a multifetal pregnancy; smoke, drink, or use drugs; are vegans, have iron-deficiency anemia, or have been diagnosed with a nutrient deficiency.

For those who need a supplement, pregnant women should take an all-in-one product, instead of individual vitamins or minerals to be sure that they are getting balanced amounts of the required nutrients. A high dose of some nutrients in a supplement, such as vitamin A, can easily reach toxic amounts and pose a risk to the fetus.

Food Safety

Because pregnancy affects the mother's immune system, pregnant women are more susceptible to the bacteria, viruses, and parasites that cause **foodborne illness** (Peles et al. 2014), which may lead to miscarriage or harm the fetus. Foods to avoid during pregnancy include soft cheese made with unpasteurized milk, raw cookie dough or cake batter, raw or undercooked fish, unpasteurized juice or cider, unpasteurized milk, raw shellfish, raw or undercooked sprouts, and undercooked eggs. A complete checklist of foods to avoid and the microorganisms that they may carry is available at: www.foodsafety.gov/risk/pregnant/chklist_pregnancy.html

Smoking, Alcohol, and Drugs

Smoking and the use of alcohol and drugs during pregnancy are associated with significant health risks to the developing fetus. Women who smoke during pregnancy have an increased risk of premature rupture of membranes associated with premature delivery. Prenatal alcohol exposure may cause miscarriage, stillbirth, and **fetal alcohol syndrome**. Illicit substance use during pregnancy also increases the chances for complications, such as **placental abruption**, early pregnancy loss, intrauterine growth retardation, late intrauterine death, placental insufficiency, postpartum hemorrhage, preeclampsia and eclampsia, and premature labor (Peles et al. 2014). Given the potential harm posed by using these substances, pregnant women are advised to avoid smoking, using alcohol, or experimenting with illicit drugs.

Adolescent Pregnancy

Pregnancy during adolescence has been associated with increased risk of miscarriage, preterm labor, low birth weight, and increased maternal and neonatal mortality (Klein 2005).

It also presents a unique set of challenges for both the mother and developing fetus, given that a pregnant teenager is still growing and developing herself. Under these circumstances, energy needs can be difficult to determine because calorie requirements vary greatly among teenagers, and are influenced by growth status, physical activity level, stage of pregnancy, and body composition.

While current recommendations for women call for an additional 340 calories per day during the second trimester, and an additional 450 calories per day during the second trimester, energy needs for pregnant teenagers may be higher. In general, pregnant adolescents should not consume less than 2,000 calories per day with the most reliable way to assess adequacy is to observe the pattern and overall amount of weight gain (Story and Hermanson 2000).

Most adolescents meet or exceed their protein requirements, which increase significantly during pregnancy. The protein DRI for adolescent females is 46 g per day, jumping to 71 g per day for pregnancy.

Fat intake should adhere to the acceptable macronutrient distribution range of 20 to 35 percent of total calories with AI of sources of linoleic and alpha-linolenic acid (essential fatty acids).

Since the pregnant teenager is still acquiring peak bone mass and needs 1,300 mg of calcium per day, it may be challenging to consume enough of the mineral through food. A prenatal supplement is advisable given the difficulties involved with not only calcium, but getting enough folate, vitamin D, iron, and zinc, and other key nutrients needed for adolescent growth.

A prenatal supplement is especially advisable for pregnant adolescents who do not regularly consume a nutritionally adequate diet, are vegans, have a multifetal pregnancy, smoke, or abuse alcohol or drugs.

Key Terms

Active Transport
The movement of molecules across a cell membrane in the direction opposite that of diffusion, that is, from an area of lower concentration to one of higher concentration. Active transport requires the assistance of a carrier protein, using energy supplied by ATP.

Adipose Tissue
A connective tissue consisting chiefly of fat cells.

Antiemetic
A substance or drug that is used to suppress nausea and vomiting.

Blastocyst
A thin-walled hollow structure in early embryonic development that contains a cluster of cells called the inner cell mass from which the embryo arises.

Cilia
Tiny hairlike projections on the surface of some cells that are capable of whipping motions to move foreign matter along.

Cognitive
Related to the mental processes of perception, memory, judgment, thinking, and reasoning.

Endocytosis
Nutrients and other molecules are engulfed by the placenta's membrane and released into the fetus' blood supply.

Estrogen
Any of a group of steroid hormones that primarily regulate the growth, development, and function of the female reproductive system. The main sources of estrogen in the body are the ovaries and the placenta.

Facilitated Diffusion
The process by which molecules diffuse across cell membranes with the help of transport proteins.

Fallopian Tube
One of a pair of long, slender ducts in the female abdomen that transport ova from the ovary to the uterus and, in fertilization, transport sperm cells from the uterus to the released ovum.

Fetal Alcohol Syndrome
A congenital syndrome caused by excessive consumption of alcohol by the mother during pregnancy, characterized by retardation of mental development and of physical growth, particularly of the skull and face of the infant.

Fetus
Unborn offspring from the end of the eighth week after conception to the moment of birth.

Foodborne Illness
Illness caused by consuming a food or beverage contaminated by disease-causing microbes, toxins, pathogens, or poisonous chemicals.

Human Chorionic Gonadotropin
A hormone produced in the human placenta that maintains the corpus luteum during pregnancy.

Human Placental Lactogen
A hormone secreted by the placenta that regulates fetal growth and metabolism; stimulates milk production and breast enlargement.

Insulin
A hormone produced by the pancreas that regulates the amount of glucose in the blood. Insulin enables cells to use glucose for energy, and when the hormone is insufficiently produced, the disease known as diabetes mellitus results.

Intrauterine Growth Restriction
Poor growth of a fetus while in the mother's womb during pregnancy.

Lactation
The secretion or production of milk by the mammary glands in female mammals after giving birth.

Neonatal
The human infant during the first month after birth.

Passive Diffusion
The process by which substances move from a region of high concentration to a region of low concentration across plasma membranes in the absence of transport proteins.

Peristalsis
The wavelike muscular contractions of the intestine or other tubular structure that propel the contents onward by alternate contraction and relaxation.

Placental Abruption
A serious pregnancy complication in which the placenta detaches from the uterus, partially or completely, depriving the baby of oxygen and nutrients; and causing heavy bleeding in the mother.

Progesterone
A steroid hormone secreted by the corpus luteum and by the placenta that acts to prepare the uterus for implantation of the fertilized ovum, to maintain pregnancy, and to promote development of the mammary glands.

Relaxin

A hormone produced by the corpus luteum during pregnancy that causes the pelvic ligaments and cervix to relax during pregnancy and delivery.

Shoulder Dystocia

A complication at birth whereby a baby's head is delivered through the vagina, but their shoulders get stuck inside the mother's body.

Stem Cell

An undifferentiated cell of a multicellular organism that is capable of giving rise to indefinitely more cells of the same type, and from which certain other kinds of cells arise by differentiation.

Umbilical Cord

The flexible cordlike structure connecting a fetus at the navel with the placenta, and containing two umbilical arteries and one vein that transports nourishment to the fetus and removes its wastes.

Zygote

A cell that is formed when an egg and sperm combine.

References

ACOG (American College of Obstetricians and Gynecologists). January 2013. "Weight Gain During pregnancy." www.acog.org/resources-And-Publications/Committee-Opinions/Committee-on-Obstetric-Practice/Weight-Gain-During-Pregnancy (accessed September 12, 2015).

Agha, M., R.A. Agha, and J. Sandell. May 2014. "Interventions to Reduce and Prevent Obesity in Pre-Conceptual and Pregnant Women: A Systematic Review and Meta-Analysis." *PLoS ONE* 9, no. 5, pp. 1–16.

American Diabetes Association. June 20, 2014. "What Is Gestational Diabetes." www.diabetes.org/diabetes-basics/gestational/what-is-gestational-diabetes.html (accessed September 14, 2015).

Austdal. M., L.H. Tangeras, R.B. Skrastad, K. Salvesen, R. Austgulen, A.C. Iversen, and T.F. Bathen. September 2015. "First Trimester Urine and Serum Metabolomics for Prediction of Preeclampsia and Gestational Hypertension: A Prospective Screening Study." *International Journal of Molecular Science* 16, no. 9, pp. 21520–38. doi:10.3390/ijms160921520

Bailey, R.L., K.P. West Jr, and R.E. Black. June 2015. "The Epidemiology of Global Micronutrient Deficiencies." *Annals of Nutrition and Metabolism* 66, suppl. 2, pp. 22–33.

Brett, K.E., Z.M. Ferraro, J. Yockell-Lelievre, A. Gruslin, and K.B. Adamo. September 2014. "Maternal-Fetal Nutrient Transport in Pregnancy Pathologies: The Role of the Placenta." *International Journal of Molecular Sciences* 15, pp. 16153–85.

Food and Drug Administration. June 10, 2014. "New Advice: Pregnant Women and Young Children Should Eat More Fish." www.fda.gov/ForConsumers/ConsumerUpdates/ucm397443.htm (accessed August 10, 2015).

Food and Nutrition Board, Institute of Medicine of the National Academies. 2005. National Agricultural Library. www.nal.usda.gov/fnic/DRI/DRI_Energy/energy_full_report.pdf

Friel, L. 2015. "Diabetes During Pregnancy." Merck Sharp & Dohme Corp. www.merckmanuals.com/home/women-s-health-issues/pregnancy-complicated-by-disease/diabetes-during-pregnancy (accessed September 14, 2015).

Institute of Medicine. 2005. "Dietary Reference Intakes: Macronutrients." http://iom.nationalacademies.org/~/media/Files/Activity%20Files/Nutrition/DRIs/New%20Material/8_Macronutrient%20Summary.pdf (accessed August 10, 2015).

Institute of Medicine. August 19, 2015. "Dietary Reference Intakes Tables and Application." http://iom.nationalacademies.org/Activities/Nutrition/SummaryDRIs/DRI-Tables.aspx (accessed September 15, 2015).

Institute of Medicine of National Academy of Sciences. May 2009. "Weight Gain During Pregnancy." https://iom.nationalacademies.org/~/media/Files/Report%20Files/2009/Weight-Gain-During-Pregnancy-Reexamining-the-Guidelines/Report%20Brief%20-%20Weight%20Gain%20During%20Pregnancy.pdf (accessed August 10, 2015).

Klein, J.D. 2005. "Adolescent Pregnancy: Current Trends and Issues." *Pediatric* 116, no. 1, pp. 281–86.

Krauss-Etschmann, S., R. Shadid, C. Campoy, E. Hoster, H. Demmelmair, M. Jiménez, A. Gil, M. Rivero, B. Veszprémi, T. Decsi, and B.V. Koletzko. May 2007. "Effects of Fish-Oil and Folate Supplementation of Pregnant Women on Maternal and Fetal Plasma Concentrations of Docosahexaenoic Acid and Eicosapentaenoic Acid: A European Randomized Multicenter Trial." *American Journal of Clinical Nutrition* 85, no. 5, pp. 1392–400.

Merck Manuals. n.d. "Stages of Development of the Fetus." www.merckmanuals.com/home/women-s-health-issues/normal-pregnancy/stages-of-development-of-the-fetus (accessed August 10, 2015).

National Institute of Child Health and Human Development. March 21, 2011. "Pregnancy and Healthy Weight." www.nichd.nih.gov/news/resources/spotlight/pages/040710-pregnancy-healthy-weight.aspx (accessed August 2, 2015).

The Nemours Foundation. May 2013. "Eating During Pregnancy." http://kidshealth.org/parent/pregnancy-center/your_pregnancy/eating-pregnancy.html (accessed August 2, 2015).

Nnam, N.M. August 2015. "Improving Maternal Nutrition for Better Pregnancy Outcomes." *Proceedings of the Nutrition Society* 74, no. 4, pp. 454–59. Epub ahead of print. PMID: 26264457.

Peles, E., A. Sason, M. Bloch, S. Maslovitz, S. Dollberg, A. Many, and M. Adelson. 2014. "The Prevalence of Alcohol, Substance and Cigarettes Exposure Among Pregnant Women with a General Hospital and the Compliance to Brief Intervention for Exposure Reduction." *Israeli Journal of Psychiatry and Related Sciences* 51, no. 4, pp. 248–57.

Procter, S.B., and C.G. Campbell. July 2014. "Position of the Academy of Nutrition and Dietetics: Nutrition and Lifestyle for a Healthy Pregnancy Outcome." *Journal of the Academy of Nutrition and Dietetics* 114, no. 7, pp. 1099–103.

Story and Hermanson. 2000. "Nutrient Needs During Adolescence and Pregnancy." In *Nutrition and the Pregnant Adolescent: A Practical Reference Guide*, eds. M. Story and J. Stang. Center for Leadership, Education, and Training in Maternal and Child Nutrition, Division of Epidemiology, School of Public Health, University of Minnesota.

U.S. Preventative Services Task Force. March 2015. "Draft Recommendation. Iron Deficiency Anemia in Pregnant Women: Screening and Supplementation." www.uspreventiveservicestaskforce.org/Page/Document/RecommendationStatementDraft/iron-deficiency-anemia-in-pregnant-women-screening-and-supplementation (accessed September 14, 2015).

Vazquez, J.C. February 2010. "Constipation, Haemorrhoids, and Heartburn in Pregnancy." *Clinical Evidence*, pp. 1–17. BMJ Publishing Group.

Wilcox, S.R. April 11, 2013. "Hyperemesis Gravidarum in Emergency Medicine." emedicine.medscape.com/article/796564-overview (accessed September 14, 2015).

Zeisel, S.H. 2006. "Choline: Critical Role During Fetal Development and Dietary Requirements in Adults." *Annual Review of Nutrition* 26, pp. 229–50.

CHAPTER 3

Feeding the Infant

Introduction

Infants will grow more rapidly during their first year after birth than at any other time in their lives, doubling their weight at six months, and tripling their weight by age one. This chapter serves as an overview of typical infant growth patterns and developmental milestones as they pertain to feeding habits and sound nutrition.

During the first few months of life, breast milk or infant formula provides all the nutrients and calories babies need, followed by the gradual introduction of solid foods, which help foster not only healthy eating habits, but help infants cultivate fine motor skills and a sense of independence through grasping and tasting new foods.

Growth

Within two days after birth, many full-term infants lose weight due to some fluid loss and passage of **meconium**. Newborns who are breastfed generally lose as much as 10 percent of their initial birth weight, while almost 5 percent of babies born vaginally and 10 percent of those born by cesarean delivery lose at least 10 percent of their initial birth weight. Typically, healthy infants will regain this lost weight within 10 to 14 days after birth (Flaherman et al. 2015), and then they should gain about 1 oz per day in the subsequent months.

At birth, an infant's head is disproportionately large compared with its body. The average head circumference of a newborn is 35 cm, which will increase by 30 percent during the first year. The skull's diameter is greater than that of the chest, and the length of the head is about a quarter of the body's total length. Also by one year, the brain doubles its birth weight, and therefore, measuring and keeping track of head circumference during this time is important for assessing brain growth (Samour, Helm, and Lang 1999).

Accurate measurements are also important for evaluating the infant's **recumbent length**, weight, and body mass index, which reflect the body's growth status, and response to any nutrition-related interventions. These measurements are routinely collected at regularly scheduled visits to the pediatrician, where they are carefully plotted on growth charts.

Growth charts provide an assessment of how the length, weight, and head circumference of an infant compare with the percentile distribution of other children at the same age for these measurements. For children age two years and older, stature is evaluated instead of recumbent length, and head circumference is no longer measured (Samour, Helm, and Lang 1999).

Growth charts are available for download from the Centers for Disease Control and Prevention (CDC) at www.cdc.gov/growthcharts/clinical_charts.htm.

The growth charts consist of a series of percentile curves that illustrate the distribution of selected body measurements in U.S. children. These percentiles categorize or rank the position of an individual child by indicating what percent of the reference population the individual would equal or exceed in terms of weight-for-age, length-for-age, and so on.

For example as explained by the CDC website,

> on the weight-for-age growth charts, a 5-year-old girl whose weight is at the 25th percentile, weighs the same or more than 25 percent of the reference population of 5-year-old girls, and weighs less than 75 percent of the 5-year-old girls in the reference population. (Centers for Disease Control and Prevention, National Center for Health Statistics 2009)

Most healthy children living in an appropriate environment will remain on the same growth curve or trajectory of growth from one year to the next. However, if there are any significant deviations in a child's growth—meaning they fall below their current curve or they jump ahead to a higher curve—it may be due to sickness or over- or undernutrition (Samour, Helm, and Lang 1999).

When plotting the growth data for infants who are premature or for those who are small at birth, it is important to make adjustments for their gestational age by subtracting the number of months of prematurity from the infant's chronological age until the child reaches two-and-a-half years of age. Then, it becomes unnecessary to make this adjustment for gestational age for most healthy premature children (Samour, Helm, and Lang 1999).

Infant Reflexes

Babies are born with a number of reflexes that sustain their feeding abilities through the first few months of life and help them consume foods in liquid form either from the breast or a bottle. These reflexes disappear by the time they are four to six months old, which is when most babies are physiologically ready to begin eating solid foods.

The "rooting" reflex prompts an infant to turn its head toward a hand when its cheek or mouth is stroked. This helps the baby find the nipple when it's time to eat. The "sucking" reflex enables a baby to start sucking when a nipple from either the breast or a bottle touches the roof of their mouth.

The "extrusion" reflex prompts a baby's tongue to thrust forward when a solid or semisolid substance is placed in its mouth, enabling the infant to reject solid food that they are not developmentally ready to eat.

Nutrient Requirements

In order to thrive, an infant needs sufficient intake of all the essential nutrients, which they can obtain through eating the right amounts and types of foods. Due to the uniquely rapid growth that occurs during the first year, the nutrient requirements per pound of body weight are proportionally higher than at any other time in the life cycle. Current nutrient recommendations for infants are based on the Dietary Reference Intakes (DRIs), developed by the Institute of Medicine's (IOM) Food and Nutrition Board. The DRIs are based on the nutrient content of foods consumed by healthy infants with normal growth patterns, the nutrient composition of breast milk, scientific research, and metabolic studies. The reference intakes for vitamins, minerals, and protein are set at levels believed to be high enough to meet the needs of most healthy infants, while energy requirements, known as the Estimated Energy Requirements (EER), are based on the needs of the average infant (United States Department of Agriculture, Food and Nutrition Service 2009a).

Energy

Infants need energy from food for activity, growth, and normal development and their calorie requirements depend on many factors, including body size and composition, metabolic rate, physical activity, size at birth, age, sex, genetic factors, and growth rate. The IOM has determined that the DRI for an infant from birth to six months is 570 kcal per day; and for an infant aged 7 to 12 months, 743 kcal per day. These numbers are based on an EER for infants and balance their energy expenditure with normal development and allows for a rate of tissue synthesis that supports good health. It is important to note that for breastfed babies, the rate of weight gain after the first three months of life may be lower than that of formula-fed infants. A general indicator of whether a baby is getting enough daily calories is their growth rate in length, weight, and head circumference (United States Department of Agriculture, Food and Nutrition Service 2009a).

Carbohydrates

Infants need adequate amounts of carbohydrate to fuel growth, body functions, and physical activity while sparing the protein required for building and repairing tissue. Adequate intake (AI) for carbohydrates from birth to six months is 60 g per day; and from 7 to 12 months the recommendation is for 95 g per day.

Lactose is the major type of carbohydrate normally consumed by young infants through their ingestion of breast milk or cow's milk-based infant formula. Infant formulas that do not contain lactose, such as those that are soy-based, provide carbohydrates in the form of sucrose, corn syrup, or corn syrup solids; while other types of specialized preparations contain carbohydrates in the form of modified corn starch, tapioca dextrin, or tapioca starch.

Some fruit juices, such as those made from prunes, apples, or pears, contain a significant amount of **sorbitol** and fructose, which infants can only absorb in limited amounts. Therefore, excessive intake of these beverages may lead to diarrhea, abdominal pain, or bloating, and so they should not be offered to infants younger than six months and limited to no more than 4 to 6 oz daily of pasteurized, 100 percent juice from a cup for infants older than six months.

Protein

High-quality protein from breast milk, infant formula, and eventually complementary foods helps babies build, maintain, and repair new tissues; and synthesize important enzymes, hormones, and antibodies. Protein can also be a potential source of energy if the infant's diet does not provide enough calories from carbohydrate or fat. Protein needs for growth per unit of body weight are initially high and then decrease with age as the child's growth rate decreases. The recommended AI for protein is 9.1 g per day from birth to six months; and the Recommended Dietary Allowance (RDA) for protein is 11 g per day from 7 to 12 months. Breast milk and infant formulas provide enough protein to meet a young infant's needs, if consumed in amounts necessary to meet their energy requirements.

The amount of protein in infant formula is higher than the amounts found in breast milk, but the body does not use this source of protein as efficiently. With the introduction of complementary food in later infancy, good sources of protein, in addition to breast milk and infant formula, include meat, poultry, fish, egg yolks, cheese, yogurt, legumes; and cereals and other grain products.

Animal-based proteins contain all the essential amino acids needed, in comparison to plant foods, which contain low levels of one or more of the essential amino acids. However, when plant foods low in one essential amino acid (i.e., legumes) are eaten on the same day with another plant food that is high in that amino acid (i.e., rice), these complementary protein foods together create a complete protein source that provide all the essential amino acids.

Fats

Fats supply approximately 50 to 55 percent of the energy consumed in breast milk and infant formula, and have several important physiological functions in the body. The accumulation of stored fat provides insulation to reduce body heat loss, and also provides padding to protect the body's organs. Dietary fats enable the body absorb the fat-soluble vitamins A, D, E, and K; and they provide essential fatty acids that are required for normal brain and eye development, healthy skin and hair, and resistance to infection and disease.

The recommended AI is 31 g per day from birth to six months, and 30 g per day from age 7 to 12 months.

Both breast milk and infant formula are good sources of fats, including essential fatty acids. Food sources of fats in the older infant's diet, other than breast milk and infant formula, include meats, dairy products, egg yolks, and any fats or oils added to home-prepared foods. There are no current restrictions on cholesterol intake for infants.

Vitamins and Minerals

Vitamin D

Vitamin D is necessary for the proper absorption and utilization of calcium in the body. The skin synthesizes vitamin D through its exposure to ultraviolet light from the sun. Therefore, the amount of vitamin D required by an infant depends on how much exposure the infant gets to sunlight. The major sources of dietary vitamin D in the United States include fortified milk products, such as milk-based infant formulas as well as fish, liver, and egg yolks.

Since breast milk contains a small amount of vitamin D, the American Academy of Pediatrics (AAP) recommends that all healthy infants have a minimum intake of 10 μg (400 IU) of Vitamin D per day during the first two months of life to prevent rickets and vitamin D deficiency. Premature and dark-skinned infants and infants with limited sunlight exposure are especially at risk of vitamin D deficiency. The AAP also recommends a supplement of 10 μg per day for all breastfed infants unless they are weaned and receiving at least 500 mL per day of vitamin D-fortified infant formula (United States Department of Agriculture, Food and Nutrition Service 2009a).

Vitamin A

Both breast milk and infant formula are major food sources of vitamin A, as are certain complementary foods, such as egg yolks, yellow and dark green leafy vegetables and fruits, and liver. Vitamin A deficiency is rare in the United States, but is pervasive in developing countries. Deficiency can lead to eye damage, poor growth, loss of appetite, and increased susceptibility to infections. The AI for infants from birth to six months is 400 µg RAEs per day, and 500 µg RAEs from 7 to 12 months.

Vitamin C

Breast milk and infant formulas are excellent sources of vitamin C, which helps to maintain capillaries, bones, and teeth; heal wounds; promote resistance to infections; and enhances the absorption of iron. Other dietary sources include vegetables such as tomatoes, cabbage, and potatoes; fruits, such as oranges, grapefruit, papaya, cantaloupe, and strawberries; and infant and regular fruit and vegetable juices naturally high in or fortified with vitamin C. Regular cow's milk, evaporated milk, and goat's milk contain very little vitamin C. The AI is 40 mg per day from birth to six months, and 50 mg per day from 7 to 12 months.

Vitamin B12

Vitamin B12 is important for healthy red blood cells, and the maintenance and functioning of the nervous system. After birth, an infant's vitamin B12 reserves generally last for about eight months. Infant formula is a major food source of vitamin B12. Babies who consume enough breast milk from mothers with adequate vitamin B12 stores can meet their needs. Complementary foods such as meat, egg yolks, and dairy products are also good sources. However, infants of breastfeeding mothers who follow strict vegetarian or vegan diets or eat very few dairy products, meat, or eggs are at risk for developing vitamin B12 deficiency. Signs of deficiency include **failure to thrive**, movement disorders, delayed development, and **megaloblastic anemia.** The IOM recommends that infants of vegan mothers be supplemented with vitamin B12 at the AI for age (zero to six months, 0.4 µg per day; 7 to 12 months, 0.5 µg per day).

Folate

Folate, or its synthetic form folic acid, is a water-soluble B-vitamin needed for proper cell division, healthy red blood cells, and the formation of genetic material. Folate occurs naturally in foods, such as green leafy vegetables, oranges, cantaloupe, whole grain products, legumes, lean beef, egg yolks, and liver, while folic acid is available from fortified or enriched grain products and dietary supplements. Young infants can obtain adequate amounts of folate from breast milk or infant formula. The AI is 65 µg per day of dietary folate equivalents (DFEs) from birth to six months, and 80 µg DFEs per day from 7 to 12 months.

Iron

Iron is a trace mineral that is a vital component of hemoglobin, the part of red blood cells that carry oxygen, and is necessary for the proper functioning of many enzymes in the body. Infants need iron for the proper formation of healthy red blood cells and the prevention of iron-deficiency anemia, a condition associated with cognitive impairment and poor academic performance. Most full-term infants are born with adequate iron reserves that become depleted at about four to six months of age.

Good dietary sources of iron for infants include breast milk, infant formula, meat, liver, legumes, whole-grain breads, cereals, fortified or enriched grain products, and dark green vegetables. Dietary iron exists in two major forms: heme iron, which is found mainly in animal-based food, such as red meat, liver, poultry and fish; it is the most absorbable form and nonheme iron, which is found in breast milk, infant formula, iron-fortified breads, cereals or other grain products, legumes, and vegetables. Foods that are rich in vitamin C enhance the absorption of nonheme iron; therefore, it is advisable to offer a good source of vitamin C with the same meal that contains plant-based iron.

Starting at four to six months of age, the AAP recommends that full-term, breastfed infants receive a supplemental source of iron preferably from complementary foods, such as iron-fortified infant cereal or meats. If a full-term, breastfed infant is unable to consume sufficient iron from dietary sources after six months of age, an oral iron supplement is recommended (United States Department of Agriculture, Food and Nutrition Service 2009a).

For full-term infants, caregivers should provide only iron-fortified infant formula (including soy-based formulas) during the first year of life. Cow's milk, goat's milk, and soy-based beverages, such as soy milk, do not contain adequate amounts of iron (United States Department of Agriculture, Food and Nutrition Service 2009c).

Calcium

Calcium is a major mineral that plays an important role in the development of bones and teeth, blood clotting, and the maintenance of healthy nerves and muscles. Both breast milk and formula are good sources of calcium for a young infant, while older babies can get additional calcium from complementary foods such as yogurt, cheese, fortified or enriched grain products, certain green leafy vegetables like collards and turnip greens, and also tofu, if made with calcium sulfate. Infants who are not breast fed and are on a strict vegetarian or vegan diet are at risk for calcium deficiency; therefore, caregivers are advised to use soy-based infant formulas, which are fortified with calcium. The AI from birth to six months is 210 mg per day, and 270 mg per day from 7 to 12 months.

Zinc

Zinc is a trace mineral that is a component of many enzymes in the body and is therefore involved in most metabolic processes. It is also important for wound healing, blood formation, general growth and maintenance of all tissues, taste perception, and proper immune function. Both breast milk and infant formula are good sources of zinc for the first six months of life. Other good dietary sources include meat, poultry, liver, egg yolks, cheese, yogurt, legumes, and whole-grain breads, cereals, and other fortified or enriched grain products. The AI for infants from birth to six months is 2 mg per day; the RDA from 7to 12 months is 3 mg per day.

Fluoride

Fluoride is not considered to be an essential nutrient, but when consumed in adequate amounts, it decreases the risk of developing tooth decay. Fluoride is incorporated into the mineral portion of the teeth, making them stronger and more resistant to decay. Small amounts of the mineral are found in varying concentrations in water supplies, and in plant and animal foods. The major dietary sources for infants are fluoridated water and infant formulas made with fluoridated water. Many communities and municipalities add fluoride to local water supplies if they are naturally low in the mineral. Most public water supplies are fluoridated to provide 0.7 to 1.2 ppm of fluoride. The majority of bottled waters do not contain adequate amounts of fluoride.

The AAP, the American Academy of Pediatric Dentistry, and the CDC recommend no fluoride supplementation for infants less than six months old. Breast milk contains little fluoride even in areas with fluoridated water. Since fluoride intake during the first six months does not affect the development of tooth decay, supplementation is not necessary. The amount of fluoride in concentrated or powdered infant formula depends on the amount of fluoride in the water used for preparing it.

For infants older than six months, whose public drinking water does not contain adequate concentrations of fluoride, a supplement is recommended in the form of fluoride drops—but it is essential to give only the amount prescribed. An excessive amount of fluoride consumed over time may cause staining or "mottling" of the teeth, a condition known as **fluorosis**.

Water

Up until complementary foods are introduced, the water requirements of healthy infants can be met exclusively through adequate amounts of breast milk or properly reconstituted infant formula. However, an infant may not be getting enough water if: the prepared infant formula is too concentrated because insufficient water is being added; the infant consumes much less infant formula or breast milk than usual because of illness; the infant is vomiting or has diarrhea or a fever; the infant consuming high-protein or salty foods, which because of their high **renal solute load**, requires more water for proper metabolism. When these foods are introduced, a baby will require about 4 to 8 oz of additional water per day. Typical signs of dehydration include: a reduced amount of urine, which is also dark yellow in color; dry membranes in the mouth; absence of tears when crying; sunken eyes; and restlessness, irritability, or lethargy (United States Department of Agriculture, Food and Nutrition Service 2009a).

Breastfeeding

The AAP recommends,

> exclusive breastfeeding for about the first six months of a baby's life, followed by breastfeeding in combination with the introduction of complementary foods until at least 12 months of age, and continuation of breastfeeding for as long as mutually desired by mother and baby. (American Academy of Pediatrics 2012)

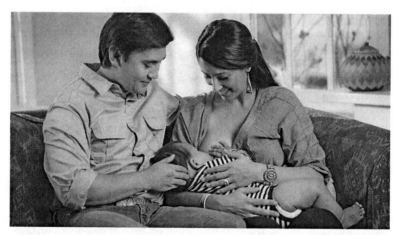

Source: https://wicworks.fns.usda.gov/nal_web/wicworks//resources/WICImages/Image33-300DPI.tif

In 2011, 79 percent of newborn infants started to breastfeed. However, that percentage declined to 49 percent at six months, and then dropped to 22 percent at 12 months (Centers for Disease Control and Prevention 2014).

Health experts consider breast milk to be the optimal food for infant growth and development because it provides the right balance of nutrients in a highly digestible and absorbable form. About 80 percent of protein in colostrum (the initial fluid from the breast) is the easily digested whey, while the remaining 20 percent is the curd-forming casein. The whey-to-casein ratio makes human milk ideal for the immature digestive tracts of young infants. In contrast, casein is the main protein in cow's milk, which makes it more difficult for infants to digest. Moreover, infants should never be given cow's milk during the first year of life because the renal solute load is too high for their immature kidneys to process, and it also causes tiny bleeds within the gastrointestinal tract (United States Department of Agriculture, Food and Nutrition Service 2009b).

Generally, the vitamin content of human milk reflects maternal intake. A well-nourished mother produces milk that contains ample amounts of most vitamins and minerals. However, many health care practitioners advise new mothers to continue taking prenatal supplements during lactation. The two vitamins that may be low in human milk are vitamin B12 and vitamin D. Because vitamin D content of human milk is reflective of the mother's sun exposure and dietary intake, amounts of the micronutrient in breast milk can vary widely. Therefore, breastfed infants should be given 10 μg of supplemental vitamin D each day.

The Physiology of Breast Milk Production

Soon after birth, the mother's level of progesterone and estrogen starts to drop, triggering the release of the hormone **prolactin**, which stimulates milk production in the breasts. Meanwhile, the brain's pituitary gland secretes another hormone called **oxytocin**, which signals the tiny muscles surrounding the **mammary glands**, located in the breast tissue to contract and release milk into a collection of ducts that are composed of alveoli—cavities within the duct that are lined with milk-producing cells.

The milk drains into an area near the nipple, and comes out of the breasts through small pores. The release of milk from the breast is known as the **let-down reflex or milk ejection reflex.**

The milk-producing cells manufacture lactose, proteins, and some fatty acids that will be incorporated into the milk and they also draw vitamins and minerals from the mother's blood and assimilate these nutrients as well. Therefore, the quality of the milk is influenced by the mother's dietary intake and nutritional status.

During the first three to four days **postpartum**, the mother's breasts secrete a thick, high-calorie, yellow-colored fluid known as **colostrum**, which is concentrated with nutrients and other substances that are highly beneficial to the infant, and also aids the passage of meconium. For this reason, even if a mother plans to bottle-feed using infant formula, it is advisable to encourage her to breastfeed for the first few days, so her baby can benefit from the health-supporting components of colostrum.

Colostrum contains

- high concentrations of easily digested protein,
- antibodies, such as secretory immunoglobulin A (sIgA), that defend the infant against bacteria and viruses, and
- hormonal components that promote the maturation of the gastrointestinal tract.

By the end of the first postpartum week, the breasts start producing transitional milk, which is a combination of colostrum and mature milk. After about two weeks, all of the milk that is produced is considered to be mature and contains higher amounts of fat, carbohydrates, minerals, and vitamins—a physiologic adaptation to the increased needs of a growing infant.

At the beginning of a breastfeeding session the mother first produces **foremilk**, which is low in fat. As the infant continues to nurse, the fat content of the milk gradually increases. The higher fat content of this **hindmilk** may make the baby feel satisfied and, as a result, discontinue feeding. Mothers should make sure the baby drains one breast before moving to the second, about 10 to 15 minutes for each. Babies who do not nurse long enough to receive the hindmilk may become hungry soon afterward.

Weight gain is the most important indicator of whether an infant is receiving sufficient milk and breastfeeding effectively. Other indicators include whether or not the baby is breastfeeding frequently and is satisfied after each feeding; can be heard swallowing consistently while breastfeeding; and has a lot of wet and soiled diapers, with pale yellow urine. During the first three to five days of life, the infant should have at least four to eight wet and three soiled diapers per day. After that, the baby should have six or more wet and three to four soiled diapers per day by five to seven days of age. After six weeks, the number of bowel movements can vary from less than once a day to several (United States Department of Agriculture, Food and Nutrition Service 2009b).

Typically, breastfeeding mothers produce about three cups of milk per day; however, milk production does rely on a physiologically-based system of supply and demand. The baby's continuing rhythm of need establishes feedings, usually about every two to three hours in the first few weeks after birth. The more a baby nurses at the nipple, the more milk is produced. However, if milk is not fully removed from the breasts, its production eventually stops. When the infant is latched onto the breast correctly, special nerve endings signal the brain to release milk-producing hormones. The amount of time an infant spends at the breast is not a guarantee that milk is being removed, because some babies are more efficient at consuming milk than others, or are latched on incorrectly so that they are getting a small amount.

To help establish a good supply, milk can be removed with a breast pump and immediately refrigerated for use within 48 hours. Otherwise, it should be frozen right away, and later thawed in warm water, but not microwaved. Refrigerated breast milk that is not used within 96 hours should be discarded (Texas Department of State Health Services 2005).

Benefits of Breast Feeding for Both Infant and Mother

Many studies suggest that exclusive breastfeeding for a period of time confers important health benefits to both the baby and the mother. Some studies indicate that breastfeeding is associated with slightly enhanced performance on tests of cognitive development (Turk et al. 2013). Because of the **immunological factors** found in breast milk, exclusive breastfeeding for three months or longer appears to be associated with a lower incidence of infant diarrhea, respiratory infections, ear infections, early childhood asthma, and **atopic dermatitis** (Turk et al. 2013) compared with formula-fed infants.

Exclusive breastfeeding may also provide many benefits for the mother. The oxytocin that is secreted by the mother's body helps shrink the uterus to its pre-pregnancy size; nursing also stimulates the release of the hormone prolactin that helps the mother feel relaxed. Some studies indicate that mothers who breastfeed their babies have lower risks of breast and ovarian cancers (Turk et al. 2013).

Breastfeeding may also be more convenient than using infant formula, because human milk is readily available and there is no need to purchase cans of formula, mix and warm preparations, or wash bottles. It is also less expensive—formula can be costly to purchase.

Breastfeeding and Maternal Diet

During lactation, a nursing mother has increased energy needs, and requires about 330 additional calories per day during the first six months of breastfeeding, and 400 additional calories per day thereafter. No special foods are necessary to maintain milk production; however, a woman should follow a nutritious and balanced diet, as well as drink fluids every time her infant nurses to help stay hydrated and to maintain an adequate milk volume.

Fortunately, there are very few contraindications to breastfeeding; however, there are certain situations where breastfeeding is not recommended including (Centers for Disease Control and Prevention 2015), when a mother

- has HIV,
- is taking antiretroviral medications,
- has active tuberculosis,
- is using illicit drugs,

- is taking prescribed cancer chemotherapy agents, and
- is undergoing radiation therapy.

Throughout lactation, a nursing mother should limit her intake of alcohol and caffeine, and should be counseled on smoking cessation programs if she smokes. Nipples that have been pierced are not a contraindication for breastfeeding, but all jewelry must be removed prior to nursing to avoid a choking hazard. Mothers who have gone through breast augmentation surgery and have silicone or saline implants can safely breastfeed (New York States Department of Health 2010). In addition, she should also check with her health care provider before using any medications, including those bought over-the-counter and herbal products, because many of these substances can be transmitted from the mother's bloodstream into the breast milk.

Infant Formula

For mothers who decide not to breastfeed their babies, commercially prepared, iron-fortified infant formulas are safe and nutritious alternatives that are manufactured under sterile conditions and approximate a mother's milk content (see Table 2.1 for a comparison of standard formula with breast milk). Just as with breast milk that has been pumped and placed in a bottle, formula can be fed to a baby by either parent or another caregiver, which allows other people to enjoy the feeding process and bond with the baby. Another convenience of bottle feeding is that the mother does not have to dedicate time to pumping or rearrange her work schedule and other activities around the baby's feeding schedule. She also does not have to worry about the food and beverages she consumes and how they may impact her baby. Because formula is digested more slowly than breast milk, babies typically can go longer between feedings, which initially is about every three to four hours.

On the other hand, infant formula does not contain any of the antibodies found in breast milk, so it does not provide the added level of protection against infections. In addition, formula feeding requires organizing and maintaining feeding supplies, such as bottles, nipples, and bottle warmers, as well as careful preparation with adequate amounts of clean, sterile water. However, with proper planning, routine formula feeding can be quite manageable. To access and print out a formula preparation checklist, visit www.dhs.state.il.us/OneNetLibrary/27897/documents/Brochures/4604.pdf.

Types of Formula

Commercial infant formulas are available as powders or concentrated liquids, which should ideally be prepared with fluoridated water; and also as pre-diluted or ready-to-feed liquids that do not contain fluoride, in which case supplemental drops should be used after the first six months.

These days, there are not only formulas created for healthy full-term infants, but many specialized ones created to address specific medical issues related to preterm births, metabolic disorders, and milk-protein intolerances. However, the most common formulas for healthy, full-term infants include iron-fortified cow's milk or soy-based products. Formulas that are made from modified cow's milk have added carbohydrate in the form of lactose, vegetable oils, as well as vitamins and minerals.

A true lactose-intolerance in infants is rare though a baby may experience transient lactose intolerance following acute diarrhea. Typically, switching to a lactose-free infant formula is not necessary because enzyme activity resumes very quickly (United States Department of Agriculture, Food and Nutrition Service 2009c). For infants who do have a documented lactose intolerance, there are several cow's milk-based formulas and soy-based formulas that are lactose-free.

For a protein source, casein is the predominant form in cow's milk, while whey protein is the predominant form in breast milk; therefore the amino acid profile in infant formula is significantly different from that in breast milk.

Soy-based infant formulas contain soy protein isolate made from soybean solids as the protein source, vegetable oils as the fat source, added carbohydrate in the form of sucrose or corn syrup solids, and vitamins and minerals. They are also fortified with the essential amino acid methionine, which is found in very low quantities in soybeans.

If an infant has an allergy or intolerance related to milk or soy protein, a number of products are available that contain partially **hydrolyzed**, extensively hydrolyzed protein, or free amino acids, which are derived from cow's milk, but the proteins are broken down into smaller chains, making them less **allergenic**. These formulas are generally well-tolerated by the vast majority of infants (United States Department of Agriculture, Food and Nutrition Service 2009c).

Given the growing body of research on the benefits of essential fatty acids to healthy eye and brain development, many formula manufacturers now include long-chain polyunsaturated fatty acids, in the form of omega-6 arachidonic acid (ARA) and omega-3 docosahexaenonic acid (DHA) in their products. Table 3.1 compares the macronutrient content of standard milk-based infant formulas with breast milk.

Introduction of Complementary Foods

Babies are generally ready to start eating complementary or solid foods by four to six months of age (bearing in mind that the AAP and the World Health Organization recommend exclusive breastfeeding of healthy full-term infants for the first six months of life). Infants do not need to eat solid foods for nutritional purposes earlier than four months, and their extrusion reflex makes feeding solids more difficult. Each baby's readiness for complementary foods depends on their level of development. There are several behavioral signs that signal physiological readiness:

- Ability to sit up with good head control
- Opening the mouth when presented with food
- Attempting to grab food
- Continuing to act hungry after breast or formula feeding

Starting solids is a gradual process that only needs to begin with a couple of spoonfuls of food mixed with some breast milk or formula into a thin consistency, and used as a complement to the child's long established feeding routine, not an immediate replacement of it. Since most breastfed babies have diminishing iron reserves by six months of age, foods that are rich in iron are good first choices. Pureed meats, such as turkey, chicken,

Table 3.1 Comparison of standard milk-based infant formulas and breast milk

	Enfamil, Enfamil LIPIL	Good Start essentials	Similac, Similac Advance	Bright Beginnings, Store brands	Breastmilk (mature)
Protein	Reduced-mineral whey, nonfat milk	Reduced-mineral whey, nonfat milk	Nonfat milk, whey-protein concentrate	Nonfat milk, Whey-protein concentrate	Human milk
Whey: Casein	60:40	60:40	52:48	60:40	80:20
% of Calories	9	9	8	9	6
Fat	Palm olein; soy, coconut, and high-oleic sunflower oils	Palm olein; soy, coconut, and high-oleic safflower oils	High-oleic safflower, coconut, and soy oils	Palm oil—palm olein; high oleic safflower or sunflower, coconut, and soy oils	Human milk fat
% of Calories	48	46	49	48	52
Carbohydrates	Lactose	Lactose	Lactose	Lactose	Lactose
% of Calories	44	45	43	43	42

Source: Texas Department of State Health Services (2005).

and beef, provide high-quality protein, iron, and zinc. Iron-fortified single-grain infant cereal, such as rice cereal and oatmeal, are other good introductory solid foods, because of their iron content, nonallergenic properties, and easy digestibility.

In order to identify any foods that a baby may be allergic to, it is advisable to introduce only one new, single-ingredient food per week and watch for reactions, such as a rash, diarrhea, or vomiting. For this reason, when starting infant cereal, it is important to carefully read the label to make sure that the cereal is a single-ingredient product and is not mixed with other foods, such as added fruit, milk, or yogurt solids. Once the baby is used to the taste and texture, the caregiver can offer more and thicker servings. The choices can be gradually expanded to offer mashed or strained fruit, and pureed vegetables. Caregivers should never put baby cereal or other foods in a bottle as it presents a choking hazard.

A balanced variety of foods each day could include the following:

- Breast milk or formula
- Pureed meats
- Infant cereal
- Pureed vegetables
- Strained fruits
- Mashed eggs
- Pureed fish (be sure to inspect for small bones)

Once the baby can sit up and bring its hands or an object to its mouth, they can try finger foods and practice feeding themselves. Soft, easy-to-swallow pieces of

- banana,
- scrambled eggs,
- soft-cooked pasta,
- finely chopped, well-cooked chicken, and
- well-cooked carrots, peas, and potatoes.

Fresh foods should be cooked with no added salt or seasoning.

Foods to Avoid

A child should be able to easily bite and chew foods. It is important to avoid foods that do not fully dissolve or break apart with chewing. Small pieces can obstruct airways; or be aspirated, causing pneumonia and other complications. Do not feed an infant foods that are round and firm, slippery, sticky, or cut in large chunks, since these foods may cause choking.

In addition, do not serve an infant the following:

- Nuts and seeds
- Raw carrots and celery
- Raw peeled apple and pear slices
- Unpeeled fruits and vegetables
- Whole beans
- Whole kernel corn
- Cherry tomatoes
- Whole grapes
- Berries
- Cherries with pits
- Raisins, dates and other dried fruits
- Large chunks of cheese or meat (especially tough meats)
- Hot dogs
- Peanuts
- Peanut butter
- Adult dry cereal
- Popcorn
- Chips
- Pretzels
- Pickles
- Whole olives
- Marshmallows (regular or miniature)
- Hard candies
- Gel or gummy candies
- Jelly beans
- Taffy
- Caramels

- Cough drops
- Chewing gum

Source: Clemson Cooperative Extension (2008).

Key terms

Allergenic
Having the capacity to induce an allergy.

Alveoli
Tiny, milk-producing sacs arranged in clusters throughout the breasts.

Atopic Dermatitis
An inflammatory skin disease, characterized by areas of severe itching, redness, and scaling.

Colostrum
The milk produced in the first two to three days after the baby is born, which is higher in protein and lower in lactose than milk produced after a milk supply is established.

Failure-to-Thrive
A condition in which a child's weight or rate of weight gain is significantly below that of other children of similar age and gender.

Fluorosis
A chronic condition caused by excessive intake of fluoride, characterized by discoloration and pitting of the teeth.

Foremilk
Breast milk at the beginning of a feeding, which has a lower fat content than the milk produced toward the end of a feeding.

Hindmilk
The breast milk at the end of a feeding, which has a higher fat content than the milk produced at the beginning of a feeding.

Hydrolyzed
Break down of a compound by chemical reaction with water.

Immunological Factors
Biologically active substances whose activities affect or play a role in the functioning of the immune system.

Let-Down Reflex or Milk Ejection Reflex
An involuntary reflex in which the breasts push out or "let down" the milk.

Mammary Gland
The source of milk for offspring, also commonly called the breast. The presence of mammary glands is a characteristic of mammals.

Meconium
The dark green substance forming the first feces of a newborn infant.

Megaloblastic Anemia
A blood disorder marked by the appearance of very large red blood cells which carry inadequate amounts of oxygen.

Oxytocin
A hormone released by the pituitary gland that triggers uterine contractions during labor, and stimulates the ejection of milk into the breast ducts.

Postpartum
The period beginning immediately after the birth of a child and extending for about six weeks.

Prolactin
A hormone necessary for milk production.

Recumbent Length
The body length of an infant measured while the child is lying down on a horizontal scale.

Renal Solute Load
All solutes (substances) that require excretion by the kidneys.

Sorbitol
A sugar alcohol with a sweet taste, which the human body metabolizes slowly. Used as a sweetener in food products.

References

American Academy of Pediatrics. February 27, 2012. "AAP Reaffirms Breastfeeding Guidelines." www.aap.org/en-us/about-the-aap/aap-press-room/pages/aap-reaffirms-breastfeeding-guidelines.aspx (accessed September 14, 2015).

American Academy of Pediatrics. August 20, 2015. "Switching to Solid Foods." www.healthychildren.org/English/ages-stages/baby/feeding-nutrition/pages/Switching-To-Solid-Foods.aspx (accessed September 10, 2015).

Centers for Disease Control and Prevention. June 17, 2015. "When Should a Mother Avoid Breastfeeding?" www.cdc.gov/breastfeeding/disease/ (accessed September 20, 2015).

Centers for Disease Control and Prevention. 2014. "Prevalence of Breastfeeding in the United States." www.cdc.gov/breastfeeding/pdf/2014breastfeedingreportcard.pdf (accessed September 10, 2015).

Centers for Disease Control and Prevention, National Center for Health Statistics. August 4, 2009. "CDC Growth Charts: United States." www.cdc.gov/growthcharts/background.htm (accessed September 18, 2015).

Clemson Cooperative Extension. October 2008. "Introducing Solid Foods to Infants." Food Science and Human Nutrition Department, Cleson University, South Carolina. www.clemson.edu/extension/hgic

Flaherman, V.J., E.W. Schaefer, M.W. Kuzniewicz, S.X. Li, E.M. Walsh, and I.M. Paul. January 2015. "Early Weight Loss Nomograms for Exclusively Breastfed Newborns." *Pediatrics* 135, no. 1, pp. e16–23.

New York States Department of Health. July 2010. "Breastfeeding Pocket Guide for Health Care Providers." www.health.ny.gov/publications/2963/ (accessed September 10, 2015).

Samour, P.Q., K.K. Helm, and C.E. Lang. 1999. "Physical Growth and Development." In *Handbook of Pediatric Nutrition*, eds. W.C. Chumlea and S.S. Guo, 3–14, 2nd ed. Gaithersburg, MD: Aspen Publishers, Inc.

Texas Department of State Health Services. January 2005. "Basic Infant Formula Module." Nutrition Services Section. Nutrition Education. Clinic Services Unit. http://webcache.googleusercontent.com/search?q=cache:r8ZkTKr9PtcJ:www.dshs.state.tx.us/wichd/tng/Linked-Files/Training-Materials/PDF/Basic-Infant-Formula+&cd=1&hl=en&ct=clnk&gl=us

Turck, D., M. Vidailhet, A. Bocquet, J.L. Bresson, A. Briend, J.P. Chouraqui, D. Darmaun, C. Dupont, M.L. Frelut, J.P. Girardet, O. Goulet, R. Hankard, D. Rieu, and U. Simeoni. November 2013. "Breastfeeding:Health Benefits for Child and Mother." *Archives of Pediatrics and Adolescent Medicine* 20, Suppl. 2, pp. S29–48.

United States Department of Agriculture, Food and Nutrition Service. March 2009a. "Chapter 1: Nutritional Needs of Infants." *Infant Nutrition and Feeding: A Guide for Use in the WIC and CSF Programs.* www.nal.usda.gov/wicworks/Topics/FG/Chapter1_NutritionalNeeds.pdf

United States Department of Agriculture, Food and Nutrition Service. March 2009b. "Chapter 3: Breastfeeding." *Infant Nutrition and Feeding: A Guide for Use in the WIC and CSF Programs.* www.nal.usda.gov/wicworks/Topics/FG/Chapter3_Breastfeeding.pdf

United States Department of Agriculture, Food and Nutrition Service. March 2009c. "Chapter 4: Infant Formula Feeding." *Infant Nutrition and Feeding: A Guide for Use in the WIC and CSF Programs.* www.nal.usda.gov/wicworks/Topics/FG/Chapter4_InfantFormulaFeeding.pdf

CHAPTER 4

Early and Middle Childhood

Introduction

The years spanning early and middle childhood are a critical time during which children learn about and establish healthy eating habits, as well as cultivate their attitudes toward food and the food choices they make for themselves. These years are a period of tremendous cognitive and physical development, presenting children, and their caregivers, countless "teachable moments" on which to build a foundation for life-long health and well-being.

The life stage covered here addresses ages two to six, which are commonly known as the "preschool" years, as well as ages 6 to 12, which are referred to as the "middle school" years. This chapter explores the growth patterns, developmental milestones, and nutrient requirements that support the vast physical and intellectual change that unfolds at this time. It also addresses the environmental and behavioral factors contributing to the current epidemic of childhood obesity that now afflicts almost 20 percent of school-aged children in the United States.

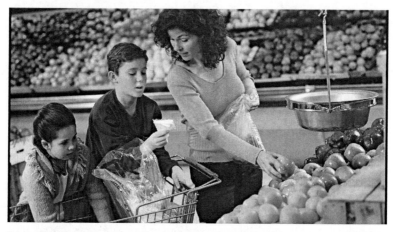

Source: https://snaped.fns.usda.gov/woman-children-shopping-fruit-2

Growth and Body Mass Index

Following the period of rapid growth during infancy, whereby a baby reaches triple its birth weight by the first year, toddlers and young children experience a significant slowdown in **growth velocity**. Generally, children have widely varying and erratic growth patterns that involve spurts in height and weight that are followed by periods of little to no growth. At the same time, children's nutrient needs and appetites typically correspond with their changes in growth rate; waxing and waning in accordance with their growth spurts (Samour, Helm, and Lang 1999).

Growth is one of the most important indicators of good health and adequate nutritional intake in children. Between ages one to three, most healthy children gain about three pounds. From ages three to six, they gain four to five pounds per year, and grow about 2 to 3 in. in height. From ages 6 to 12, height, weight, and build vary significantly from child to child. At the same time, they begin to develop a sense of **body image**, starting at about age six (U.S. National Library of Medicine 2014).

As discussed in Chapter 3, the best way to assess adequate growth in children is by using weight-for-age and height-for-age growth charts to track an individual's trajectory and placement on a percentile curve. Another useful **anthropometric** measure is pediatric body mass index (BMI).

BMI is a person's weight in kilograms divided by the square of height in meters, and is often (but not always) an indicator of body fatness. It is not a direct measurement of fat (and can be misleading if an individual's weight is mostly due to muscularity), but research has shown that BMI measurements often do correlate with other direct measurements of **adiposity**, such as **skinfold thickness**, and **bioelectrical impedance**. It is an inexpensive, quick, and easy way to screen for possible weight issues that may lead to health problems.

BMI is measured differently in adults than in children. For children, BMI is evaluated using age- and gender-specific charts that take into account the different growth patterns for each sex. Weight and the amount of fat in the body differ for boys and girls, and both weight and percentage body fat change as children grow taller and older. Therefore, throughout childhood, BMI is a measurement that does not remain constant, because height is used to calculate it. So, plotting BMI-for-age percentiles on a growth chart is the only way to evaluate whether or not a child's weight falls within the normal range for their age.

These charts help health care providers determine how a child's BMI reading compares to those of other U.S. children of the same gender and age. These groups are divided into percentiles that reflect whether a child is at a healthy weight, underweight, overweight, or obese. Links to access the appropriate BMI charts are available below.

2 to 20 years: Boys

Body mass index-for-age percentiles

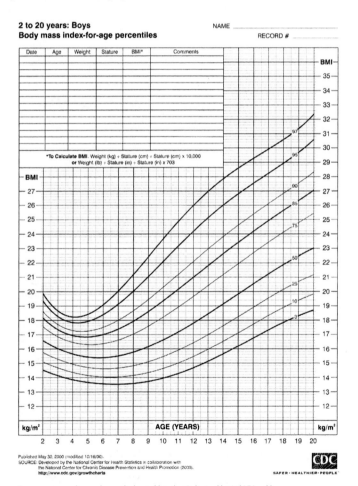

Source: www.cdc.gov/growthcharts/data/set2clinical/cj41l073.pdf

2 to 20 years: Girls

Body mass index-for-age percentiles

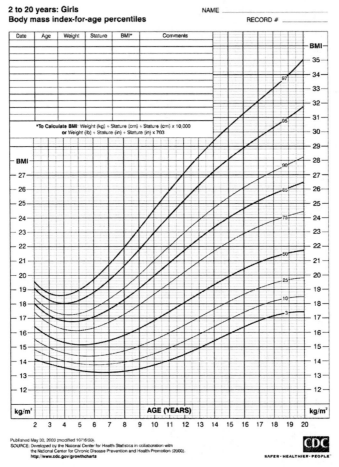

Source: www.cdc.gov/growthcharts/data/set2clinical/cj4ll074.pdf

How to Interpret the BMI Chart

Children age two and older whose BMI is:

- less than the 5th percentile are considered underweight;
- between the 5th percentile and less than the 85th percentile are at a healthy weight;

- in the 85th percentile to less than the 95th percentile are considered overweight; and
- equal to or greater than the 95th percentile are considered obese.

Another way to assess a child's growth and level of maturation is through observation of their **developmental milestones**. For example, a one year old should be able to pick up a small object using the tip of their thumb and index finger (known as the pincer grasp), enabling them to grasp and handle food. With increasing dexterity, a child will soon be able to hold a spoon or a fork. By age two, most children can communicate their needs, such as thirst and hunger. By age three, they should be able to feed themselves without much assistance.

Nutrient Requirements

During the process of transitioning from toddlerhood to school age, children's energy requirements per kilogram of body weight decrease in tandem with their slowing growth rate. However, regardless of age, energy needs throughout childhood can vary widely depending on height, weight, **basal metabolic rate** (BMR), growth, and physical activity level. Therefore, a child's calorie consumption must be adequate enough to support growth and development, and fuel their activities without the body needing to use protein stores as an energy source.

From birth through age 10 years, there is little difference in energy requirements between boys and girls. However, after about age 10, there are wider differences in calorie recommendations for each gender, because of the different age in which **puberty** begins. There is much variability in the timing and extent of the **adolescent** growth spurt as well as differences in physical activity level among children. Table 4.1 summarizes the daily energy requirements of each gender within specific age ranges. These recommendations are based on equations used for estimating average energy requirements.

Protein

During childhood, adequate protein intake is especially important for building muscles and bones, and promoting growth. In the United States,

Table 4.1 Estimated energy requirements

	Age (years)	Energy (kcal/day)
Male	1–3	1,046
	4–8	1,742
	9–13	2,279
Females	1–3	992
	4–8	1,642
	9–13	2,071

Table 4.2 Recommended dietary allowance for protein

	Age (years)	RDA for Protein (g/day)
Males	1–3	13
	4–8	19
	9–13	34
Females	1–3	13
	4–8	19
	9–13	34

protein deficiency among children is rare; however, it can occur in those who follow a strict vegan diet, suffer from severe food allergies, or are in a situation with limited access to food. Otherwise, most healthy children can easily meet their protein requirements by consuming a balanced and varied diet. Table 4.2 summarizes the daily protein requirements of children by gender and age range.

Carbohydrates

Carbohydrates are the preferred fuel source for the brain and active growing muscles. Nutrient dense choices such as whole grain cereals, brown rice, milk, starchy vegetables like potatoes, peas, corn, and yams, fruits, and legumes provide calories as well as vitamins, minerals, and fiber. Foods and beverages such as candy, cakes, cookies, soda, and juice cocktails are a source of added sugar and calories, but lacking in essential nutrients. For children ages one to three, the RDA for fiber is 19 g per day; while for children age four to eight the recommendation is 24 g per day.

Fats

Fats are nutrients in food that the body uses to build and insulate nerve and brain tissue, as well as produce hormones. Whatever fat the body does not use for fuel or building tissue gets stored in fat cells. While too much fat may lead to excessive calorie intake and adiposity, children require adequate amounts of healthy fats for normal brain and nervous system development. Dietary fats are important for good health because they

- supply fuel,
- help the body absorb the fat-soluble vitamins A, D, E, and K,
- provide the building blocks for hormones,
- insulate nervous system tissue, and
- promote **satiety**, which discourages overeating.

While for years, low-fat diets have been heavily promoted as important for weight management and cardiovascular health, some health experts believe that the importance on low-fat and no-fat foods has been overblown, and overlooks the critical role fats play in the body. For children under two years of age especially, fats should not be restricted. For children up to the age of three, the recommended intake of fats for decades was 30 to 35 percent of total calories; and from ages four and older the recommendation was 25 to 35 percent of total calories. However, in 2015 the Dietary Guidelines Advisory Committee recommended an elimination of an upper limit on total daily fat consumption and lifting restrictions on cholesterol intake (Mozaffarian and Ludwig 2015).

Vitamins and Minerals

Vitamins and minerals are essential nutrients throughout life. However, certain ones are particularly important for growth and development during childhood. For example, when children do not eat enough fruits and vegetables or fortified cereals, they are at risk for obtaining inadequate amounts of vitamins A and C. Likewise, without adequate sun exposure or consumption of fortified foods, they may not get enough vitamin D either. Vitamin A promotes normal growth and development, tissue and bone repair, and healthy skin, eyes, and immune function (see Table 1.2 in Chapter 1 for a list of major food sources). Vitamin C is necessary for healthy muscles, connective tissue, and skin. Vitamin D is important for bone and tooth formation and proper calcium absorption.

As for the B-complex vitamins, which include thiamin, niacin, ribo-flavin, and B12, if children consume a variety of foods, especially grains, cereals, meat, meat substitutes, and dairy, their needs will likely be met.

With regard to minerals, national surveys indicate that children do not get adequate amounts of calcium, which is particularly important for build-ing strong bones and teeth (see Table 1.5 in Chapter 1 for a list of major food sources). While data suggests that the average daily calcium intake of younger children exceeds recommendations, most older children do not get adequate amounts (Greer and Krebs 2006; Ogata and Hayes 2014).

Children, in particular, also need adequate amounts of iron to accom-modate their expanding blood volume during periods of rapid growth (see Table 1.7 in Chapter 1 for a list of major food sources). According to research cited by the U.S. Department of Health and Human Services, 5.3 percent of children aged three to four were iron deficient during 2005 to 2008 (U.S. Department of Health and Human Services 2020).

Food Plans

Most healthy children can obtain all the essential nutrients they need from a varied and nutrient-dense diet that includes choices from all five food groups: grains, vegetables, fruits, dairy, and protein. Table 4.3 is a summary of information from several *Daily Food Plans* based on age and calorie level available from the U.S. Department of Agriculture's (USDA) *Choose My Plate* website. To access individual food plans go to: www.choosemyplate.gov/tools-daily-food-plans.

What Is a Serving

Grains: a 1-oz serving equivalent is one slice of bread; 1 oz of ready-to-eat cereal; ½ cup of cooked rice, pasta, or cereal.

Vegetables: a serving is equivalent to one cup of raw or cooked vegetables; two cups of leafy salad greens; and one cup of 100 percent vegetable juice.

Table 4.3 *Summary of food groups and daily serving recommendations based on calorie level*

Age (years)	Calorie level	Grains	Vegetables	Fruits	Dairy	Protein
2	1,000	3 oz	1 cup	1 cup	2 cups	2 oz
3	1,200	4 oz	1 ½ cups	1 cup	2 cups	3 oz
4–5	1,400	5 oz	1 ½ cups	1 ½ cups	2 ½ cups	4 oz
6–8	1,600	5 oz	2 cups	1 ½ cups	2 ½ cups	5 oz
9–11	1,800	6 oz	2 ½ cups	1 ½ cups	3 cups	5 oz

Fruits: a serving is equivalent to one cup of raw or cooked fruit; ½ cup of dried fruit; and one cup of 100 percent fruit juice.

Dairy: one serving is equivalent to one cup of milk, yogurt, or fortified soy beverage; 1½ oz of natural cheese; and 2 oz of processed cheese.

Protein Foods: one serving is equivalent to 1 oz of lean meat, poultry, or seafood; one egg; one tablespoon of peanut butter, ¼ cup of cooked beans or peas; ½ oz of nuts or seeds.

Healthy People 2020

In recognizing that the pre- and middle school years set the stage for later health in adulthood, Healthy People 2020 (the federal government's goals for the health of the nation) added several new objectives that address nutrition-related issues throughout childhood. Many of these objectives place particular focus on weight status (Ogata and Hayes 2014), since childhood obesity has more than doubled in children and quadrupled in adolescents in the past 30 years (Centers for Disease Control and Prevention 2015a). However, based on national surveys, it appears that for some age groups, the obesity rate has at least stabilized in recent years, possibly stemming from public health efforts to reign in the epidemic (Ogata and Hayes 2014).

Some of the objectives of Healthy People 2020 related to Nutrition and Weight Status include the following:

- Increase the proportion of schools that offer nutritious foods and beverages outside of school meals.
- Increase the proportion of primary care physicians who regularly measure the BMI of their patients.
- Reduce the proportion of children and adolescents who are considered obese.
- Increase the contribution of fruits to the diets of the population aged 2 years and older.
- Increase the variety and contribution of whole grains to the diets of the population aged 2 years and older.
- Reduce consumption of calories from solid fats and added sugars in the population aged 2 years and older.

Food Safety and Young Children

Anyone at any age can acquire a **food-borne illness**, but infants and toddlers are particularly vulnerable because of their still immature immune systems that cannot fight off an infection as well as an older child. Food poisoning can happen after eating something that has been contaminated by bacteria, viruses, toxins, molds, and parasites. The symptoms generally can include but are not limited to abdominal cramps, nausea, vomiting, diarrhea, and a fever. These symptoms are especially serious for infants and toddlers because dehydration can set in very quickly and lead to weakness and an irregular heartbeat. For this reason, adequate fluid intake is the main course of treatment while waiting for symptoms to subside. Generally, carbonated drinks and beverages with a lot of sugar can make diarrhea worse, so plain tea, water, diluted fruit juices, and popsicles are preferable. A pediatrician may recommend a store-bought rehydration solution, and bland foods as tolerated, such as bananas, toast, and crackers.

The Academy of Nutrition and Dietetics (AND) recommends that parents and caregivers always avoid feeding young children:

- Unpasteurized milk or any unpasteurized dairy products
- Raw or partially cooked eggs or foods containing raw eggs
- Raw or undercooked meat and poultry
- Raw and undercooked fish or shellfish
- Unpasteurized juices
- Raw sprouts
- Honey (avoid until after the baby's first birthday because it can harbor spores of toxic bacterium that can cause botulism, a severe foodborne illness caused by a bacterium that occurs in soil). (Academy of Nutrition and Dietetics 2015)

Oral Health

Tooth decay, also known as dental caries, is the most common chronic condition that occurs during childhood. It results when bacteria colonize on tooth surfaces and subsequently metabolizes fermentable carbohydrates into acids that demineralize tooth enamel. For children, tooth decay can have serious long-term health effects, including oral pain, inadequate dietary intake, and failure-to-thrive. From 1999 to 2004, 42 percent of children age 2 to 11 had tooth decay in their primary teeth (Palmer and Gilbert 2012).

While genetics can play a role in an individual's susceptibility to tooth decay, a major environmental factor that contributes to the proliferation of dental bacteria is dietary sugar intake. Sugars are especially **pathogenic** if they are eaten very frequently and in a form that remains in the mouth for long periods of time, such as those found in sticky candy or soda that is repeatedly sipped (Segura et al. 2014).

In contrast to the effect of sugar on tooth enamel, saliva production in adequate amounts provides a buffering effect on the acid level and promotes **remineralization** of the tooth's surface. Saliva also flushes out food particles, and contains calcium and phosphate, which enhances remineralization as well (Segura et al. 2014).

Studies show that the most effective way to prevent the development of childhood tooth decay is the adequate consumption of the trace mineral fluoride, which aids tooth resistance to acid demineralization (Palmer and Gilbert 2012).

Fluoride's effectiveness is mostly seen through its **topical** application in the form of fluoridated toothpastes and mouth rinses, as well as its ingestion from fluoridated water and oral supplements (Segura et al. 2014).

There are three major ways that fluoride works to prevent the development of tooth decay. It inhibits the demineralization of tooth surfaces, enhances the remineralization process, and it inhibits bacterial enzymes from damaging tooth enamel (Segura et al. 2014).

The American Academy of Pediatrics (AAP) has made the following recommendations for the prevention of childhood tooth decay:

- Avoid putting a child to bed with a bottle.
- Limit sugary foods and drinks to mealtimes.
- Avoid carbonated, sugared beverages and juice drinks that are not 100 percent juice.
- Limit the intake of 100 percent fruit juice to no more than 4 to 6 oz per day.

- Encourage children to drink only water between meals, preferably fluoridated tap water.
- Fluoride supplements should be prescribed for children whose primary source of drinking water is deficient in fluoride.

Childhood Obesity

The epidemic of childhood obesity has become one of the most prominent global health problems of this century. The World Health Organization (WHO) has estimated that worldwide there are 43 million overweight children under the age of five (Kelishadi and Azizi-Soleiman 2014). In the United States, the percentage of children ages 6 to 11 years who are obese increased from 7 percent in 1980 to nearly 18 percent in 2012 (Centers for Disease Control and Prevention 2015a).

Pediatric obesity increases children's risk for developing high cholesterol levels, high blood pressure, as well as **prediabetes**, and eventually cardiovascular problems. They are also at greater risk for bone and joint problems, sleep disturbances, and social and psychological issues related to feeling judged and criticized by their peers, and poor self-esteem. In addition, children who are obese are more likely to be so as adults, and therefore are more likely to develop health problems such as heart disease, type 2 diabetes, stroke, **osteoarthritis**, and certain types of cancers (Centers for Disease Control and Prevention 2015a).

Fortunately, during the past decade or so, as the long-term health consequences of childhood obesity has gained more visibility, there have been significant public health initiatives throughout the United States aimed at reversing the trend. These efforts may have resulted in some successes given that the prevalence rate of childhood obesity appears to have leveled off in certain major cities. From 2003 to 2004, the obesity rate among children aged two to five was 13 percent. However, from 2011 to 2012, the prevalence of obesity among this age group dropped to 8.4 percent (Robert Wood Johnson Foundation 2015). Changes to state-level legislation that impacts schools and childcare centers, as well as comprehensive programs that integrate more physical activity and wellness policies, may be some of the factors that have led to this recent decline in obesity rates (Robert Wood Johnson Foundation 2015).

However, additional data shows that there is a concerning upward trend in the number of children with severe obesity. According to a recent study, 4 percent of children were severely obese during 1999 to 2004. By 2011 to 2012, 6 percent were severely obese (Skinner et al. 2015).

Unfortunately, the consequences of severe childhood obesity can be very serious. When compared to their moderately obese peers, children with severe obesity have a higher risk for adult obesity, early heart disease, hypertension, type 2 diabetes, **metabolic syndrome**, **fatty liver disease**, and premature death. The environmental and behavioral factors that contribute to the development of severe obesity are the same as those that promote the less severe form (Bass and Eneli 2015).

Some of the risk factors for childhood obesity include genetic susceptibility, an **obesogenic** diet high in sugar-sweetened beverages, fast-food and processed snacks, decreased physical activity, and shorter sleep duration (Brown et al. 2015).

Since many health experts view early childhood to be a critical period for habit formation, it is a crucial time to implement obesity prevention efforts (Mazarello, Ong, and Lakshman 2015). Research shows that the factors that tend to promote obesogenic diets in children aged zero to six include negative parent modeling, lack of knowledge, time constraints, using food as a reward, lack of affordability and availability of healthier food choices, and the advertising of less healthy foods to children (Mazarello, Ong, and Lakshman 2015).

Therefore, there needs to be a comprehensive approach to obesity management and prevention that encompasses environmental and behavioral influences for both children and their caregivers. Pediatricians can help prevent obesity by measuring BMI at least yearly, and providing guidance to families to encourage positive modeling behavior and the creation of home environments that promote healthy diets (Brown et al. 2015).

For children who are already overweight, a management strategy should include modified energy, fat, and sugar intake, along with increased physical activity. At the same time, it is important to monitor linear growth, as well as ensure that dietary protein intake is adequate enough to preserve **lean body mass**. The aim is to stop or slow weight gain until the child grows into an appropriate weight for their height.

An important component of any obesity prevention or weight management treatment is adequate amounts of exercise. Starting at about age 6, children should get at least 60 minutes or more of physical activity each day, as recommended by the *Physical Activity Guidelines for Americans*. Whatever exercise children participate in, they should be physical activities that kids enjoy, are appropriate for their age, and offer variety. It is also important to keep in mind that children need to engage in three types of physical work. *Aerobic* activity should make up most of their 60 or more minutes of exercise each day. This can include brisk walking or running at least three days per week. *Muscle-strengthening* activities, such as gymnastics or push-ups, are also important and should be performed at least three days per week, and then *bone-strengthening* activities, such as jumping rope or running at least three days per week as well (Centers for Disease Control and Prevention 2015b).

Key Terms

Adiposity
Consisting of or relating to animal fat stored in the fatty tissue of the body.

Adolescent
Relating to or undergoing adolescence. A young person who has undergone puberty but has not reached full maturity; a teenager.

Anthropometric
Related to human body measurements especially on a comparative basis.

Basal Metabolic Rate
Measurement of basal metabolism, which is the minimum number of calories the body uses for vital physiological activities after fasting and resting for 12 hours.

Bioelectrical Impedance
Resistance to electrical current as it travels through body fluids and tissues. Its measurement is used in body composition analysis to determine total water, lean mass, and other body components.

Body Image
An intellectual or idealized image of what one's body is or should be like, established by self-observation and by noting the reactions of others.

Developmental Milestones
Typical behaviors or physical skills seen in infants and children as they grow and develop.

Fatty Liver Disease
A condition in which an excess level of fat builds up in the liver and interferes with the organ's normal functioning. Symptoms may include fatigue and vague abdominal discomfort. If inflammation is present, symptoms may include poor appetite, nausea, weight loss, abdominal pain, and weakness.

Food-borne Illness
Illness that is caused by food contaminated with bacteria, viruses, parasites, mold, or toxins.

Growth Velocity
The rate of growth or change in growth measurements over a period of time.

Lean Body Mass
The weight of a person's body that is not body fat; including muscles, organs, and bones.

Metabolic Syndrome
A cluster of biochemical and physiological abnormalities (increased blood pressure, high blood sugar level, excess body fat around the waist, and abnormal cholesterol levels) that increase the risk of developing heart disease, stroke, and diabetes.

Obesogenic
Tending to cause obesity.

Osteoarthritis
A degeneration of the flexible tissue (joint cartilage) between the ends of bones, causing pain and stiffness.

Pathogenic
Causing or capable of causing disease.

Prediabetes
A condition in which blood sugar is high, but not high enough to be considered type 2 diabetes.

Puberty
The period during which adolescents reach sexual maturity and become capable of reproduction.

Remineralization
The restoration or return of lost mineral elements to the body, especially to bones and teeth.

Satiety
The quality or state of being fed to or beyond capacity.

Skinfold Thickness
A noninvasive, quantitative technique for determining a person's body fat composition by measuring the width of the subcutaneous (under the skin) fat with calipers at various skinfold sites on the body.

Topical
Relating to or applied on the surface of a part of the body.

References

Academy of Nutrition and Dietetics. 2015. "Food Safety Tips for Young Children." www.eatright.org/resource/homefoodsafety/safety-tips/food-poisoning/food-safety-tips-for-young-children

Bass, R., and I. Eneli. 2015. "Severe Childhood Obesity: An Under-Recognised and Growing Health Problem." *Postgraduate Medical Journal* 91, pp. 639–45.

Brown, C.L., E.E. Halvorson, G.M. Cohen, S. Lazorick, and J.A. Skelton. 2015. "Addressing Childhood Obesity: Opportunities for Prevention." *Pediatric Clinics of North America* 62, no. 5, pp. 1241–61.

Centers for Disease Control and Prevention. August 2015a. "Childhood Obesity Facts." www.cdc.gov/healthyschools/obesity/facts.htm

Centers for Disease Control and Prevention. June 4, 2015b. "How Much Physical Activity Do Children Need?" www.cdc.gov/physicalactivity/basics/children/index.htm

Greer, F.R., and N.F. Krebs. 2006. "Optimizing Bone Health and Calcium Intake of Infants, Children, and Adolescents." *Pediatrics* 117, no. 2, pp. 578–85.

Kelishadi, R., and F. Azizi-Soleiman. 2014. "Controlling Childhood Obesity: A Systematic Review on Strategies and Challenges." *Journal of Research in Medical Sciences* 19, no. 10, pp. 993–1008.

Mazarello, P.V., K.K. Ong, and R. Lakshman. 2015. "Factors Influencing Obesogenic Dietary Intake in Young Children (0–6 Years): Systematic Review of Qualitative Evidence." *British Medical Journal Open* 5, no. 9: e007396.

Mozaffarian, D., and D.S. Ludwig. 2015. "The 2015 US Dietary Guidelines. Lifting the Ban on Total Dietary Fat." *Journal of the American Medical Association* 313, no. 24, pp. 2421–22.

Ogata, B.N., and D. Hayes. 2014. "Position of the Academy of Nutrition and Dietetics: Nutrition Guidance for Healthy Children Ages 2 to 11 years." *Journal of the Academy of Nutrition and Dietetics* 114, no. 8, pp. 1257–76.

Palmer, C.A., and J.A. Gilbert. 2012. "Position of the Academy of Nutrition and Dietetics: The Impact of Fluoride and Health." *Journal of the Academy of Nutrition and Dietetics* 112, no. 9, pp. 1443–53.

Robert Wood Johnson Foundation. February 2015. "Declining Childhood Obesity Rates: Where Are We Seeing Signs of Progress?" www.rwjf.org/content/dam/farm/reports/reports/2015/rwjf417749 (accessed September 28, 2015).

Samour, P.Q., K.K. Helm, and C.E. Lang. 1999. *Handbook of Pediatric Nutrition.* Gaithersburg, MD: Aspen Publishers.

Segura, A., S. Boulter, M. Clark, R. Gereige, D.M. Krol, W. Mouradian, R. Quinonez, F. Ramos-Gomez, R. Slayton, and M.A. Keels. 2014. "Maintaining and Improving the Oral Health of Young Children." *Pediatrics* 134, no. 6, pp. 1224–29.

Skinner, A.C., E.M. Perrin, L.A. Moss, and J.A. Skelton. 2015. "Cardiometabolic Risks and Severity of Obesity in Children and Young Adults." *New England Journal of Medicine* 373, no. 14, pp. 1307–17.

U.S. Department of Health and Human Services. 2020. "Topics & Objectives. Maternal, Infant, and Child Health." Office of Disease Prevention and Health Promotion. http://www.healthypeople.gov/2020/topics-objectives/topic/maternal-infant-and-child-health

U.S. National Library of Medicine. February 26, 2014. "Normal Growth and Development." MedlinePlus. www.nlm.nih.gov/medlineplus/ency/article/002456.htm

United States Department of Agriculture. n.d. "My Daily Food Plan." www.choosemyplate.gov/tools-daily-food-plans

CHAPTER 5

Nutrition for the Adolescent

Introduction

Adolescence is a time of tremendous developmental, physical, and emotional change. In fact, with the exception of infancy, there is no other stage in the human lifecycle that involves such extensive transformation. Throughout this period, children transition from childhood to adulthood. They gain up to 50 percent of their adult body weight and 50 percent of their bone mass, attain the physical capacity to reproduce, and experience ongoing brain development.

Given such rapid growth, teenagers require adequate calories and nutrients to meet their evolving needs. This chapter explores some of the specific nutrients that are critical to this stage of life, as well as other health-related issues that affect adolescents, such as smoking and alcohol use, the existing prevalence of obesity, and problems associated with disordered eating and body image.

Growth

Adolescence is generally defined as the second decade of life. However, research indicates that the physical and **neurological** changes that typically take place during this stage may start as early as age 8 and last until age 24 (McNeely and Blanchard 2009).

During the adolescent years and at widely varying times, signs of **secondary sexual characteristics** begin to emerge as children enter the phase of *puberty*, a developmental stage that the World Health Organization (WHO) defines as "the period of life when a child experiences physical, hormonal, sexual and social changes and becomes capable of reproduction." For girls, puberty typically starts between the ages of 8 and

13; and for boys, it begins between the ages of 9 and 14 (McNeely and Blanchard 2009).

During puberty, girls experience a rapid growth spurt that often starts around age 10 and lasts for a few years. The stage of early female puberty is characterized by breast bud development, the appearance of pubic and underarm hair, increased height, menstrual onset, and widening hips. Past their mid-teen years, girls will continue to grow until they are 17 or 18 years old, but at a slower rate (McNeely and Blanchard 2009).

A pubertal growth spurt in boys usually begins one to two years after most girls and continues for three to four years. Often, boys do not complete their physical growth until about age 21. In males, secondary sexual characteristics include the emergence of pubic and underarm hair, the lengthening of the penis, an increase in height, a deepened voice, and significantly added muscle mass compared with girls (McNeely and Blanchard 2009).

For both girls and boys, puberty is triggered by the actions of hormones on various parts of the body, which are at work for several months before development becomes outwardly evident. Meanwhile, the timing of physical and cognitive changes varies throughout adolescence. Even if a teenager is adult-sized, they may not be fully developed emotionally or psychologically. On the other hand, a teenager who does not appear to have completed their growth could display more advanced reasoning and abstract thinking skills compared with their more physically developed peers of the same age (McNeely and Blanchard 2009). Table 5.1, summarizes some of the key developmental features of adolescence.

Table 5.1 Key features in adolescent development ages 10 to 19

Females	Males
Increase in body fat	Increase in muscularity
Breast growth	Increased growth of testicles and penis
Onset of menstrual periods	Deepening of voice
Increase in height and weight	Increase in height and weight
Oilier skin and hair	Oilier skin and hair
Possible appearance of acne	Possible appearance of acne
Body hair growth (underarm and pubic)	Body hair growth (underarm, pubic, facial)

Source: McNeely and Blanchard (2009).

Nutrient Requirements

Regardless of what stage of life a person is in, everyone requires the same essential nutrients in differing quantities. Teenagers in particular need key micronutrients in adequate amounts, along with sufficient levels of macronutrients to support the rapid growth and development of adolescence. Because there are such wide variations in physical size, growth velocity, and metabolic rate, there is little definitive data on what is the optimal level of nutritional and caloric intake for adolescents. Current recommendations are extrapolated from the nutritional requirements of adults and children and are based on chronological age rather than physiological level of development. Table 5.2 is a summary of information from several *Daily Food Plans* based on age and calorie level from the U.S. Department of Agriculture's *Choose My Plate* website. To access individual food plans go to: www.choosemyplate.gov/tools-daily-food-plans.

What Is a Serving

Grains: a 1-oz serving equivalent is one slice of bread; 1 oz of ready-to-eat cereal; ½ cup of cooked rice, pasta, or cereal.

Vegetables: a serving is equivalent to one cup of raw or cooked vegetables; two cups of leafy salad greens; and one cup of 100 percent vegetable juice.

Fruits: a serving is equivalent to one cup of raw or cooked fruit; ½ cup of dried fruit; and one cup of 100 percent fruit juice.

Dairy: one serving is equivalent to one cup of milk, yogurt, or fortified soy beverage; 1½ oz of natural cheese; and 2 oz of processed cheese.

Protein Foods: one serving is equivalent to 1 oz of lean meat, poultry, or seafood; one egg; one tablespoon of peanut butter, ¼ cup of cooked beans or peas; ½ oz of nuts or seeds.

Energy

The timing of growth and maturation among adolescents varies greatly and therefore the energy needs of teenagers vary as well. A teenager's calorie requirements are influenced by activity level, basal metabolic rate (BMR), and their level of lean body mass. Since adolescent boys typically

Table 5.2 Summary of food groups and daily serving recommendations based on calorie level

Age (years)	Calorie level	Grains	Vegetables	Fruits	Dairy	Protein
9–17	2,000	6 oz	2 ½ cups	2 cups	3 cups	5 ½ oz
9–17	2,200	7 oz	3 cups	2 cups	3 cups	6 oz
9–17	2,400	8 oz	3 cups	2 cups	3 cups	6 ½ oz
9–17	2,600	9 oz	3 ½	2 cups	3 cups	6 ½ oz
9–17	2,800	10 oz	3 ½	2 ½	3 cups	7 oz
9–17	3,000	10 oz	4 cups	2 ½	3 cups	7 oz

Table 5.3 EER based on light to moderate activity level

	Females 9–13 (yrs)	Females 14–18 (yrs)	Males 9–13 (yrs)	Males 14–18 (yrs)
EER (kcal)	2,071	2,368	2,279	3,152

have greater increases in height, weight, and lean body mass compared with girls, their calorie requirements are higher. However, a highly athletic female may need more calories than a sedentary male of the same age. Those adolescents participating in sports, or those who are training to build up muscle mass, may require additional energy to meet their individual needs. Given such diverse energy requirements among teenagers, the most reliable method for assessing whether an individual's calorie intake is adequate is to evaluate their height and weight, and to observe whether these measurements remain within the same growth chart percentile curves over time. Table 5.3 summarizes the estimated energy requirements (EER) of adolescents ages 9 to 18.

Carbohydrates

Carbohydrates in the form of starches and sugars provide the body with its primary source of energy. They are present in varying amounts in grains, legumes, fruits, vegetables, dairy products, and in other foods containing added sugar, such as soda and candy. Foods such as fruit, vegetables, whole grains, and legumes, are also major sources of dietary fiber, a nondigestible form of carbohydrate that contributes to both digestive and cardiovascular health, and is an important component of an overall healthy diet. The minimum recommended intake of carbohydrates for adolescents is 130 g per day; or optimally 45 to 65 percent of daily energy needs. For teenage girls, the recommended amount of fiber they need is 26 g per day; and for teenage boys younger than 14, the recommended amount is 31 g per day, and for older boys it is 38 g per day.

Protein

Every human cell contains proteins, which are the building blocks of life. Protein is found in muscle, bone, skin, and hair, and is part of the enzymes responsible for many chemical reactions in the body. It is needed for the repair and creation of cells, and is therefore critical for the growth and development of children and adolescents. The protein requirements of teenagers depends not only on how much they need to maintain their existing lean body mass, but also the amount they require to build additional mass during growth spurts. Currently, the estimated protein need for adolescents is 0.85 g per kg of body weight per day, slightly higher than that of adults. Protein requirements are highest for females at ages 11 to 14, and for males at ages 15 to 18, when growth peaks. Quality sources of animal protein include lean meats, fish, poultry, eggs, and dairy. Complementary plant sources are combinations of nuts and nut products, seeds, grains, legumes, and vegetables.

Fats

The human body requires dietary fat for normal growth, development, and optimum health. One of its major functions is as an energy reserve, but fats also contribute to normal signal transmission between cells, the structure of cellular membranes, the protection of the body's organs, and the proper absorption of the fat-soluble vitamins. The energy obtained from fat plays an important role for both high intensity and endurance sports, and serves as the primary fuel for physical activities that are of low intensity and long duration.

To date, recommendations suggest that children over the age of two years consume no more than 25 to 35 percent of calories from fat, with no more than 10 percent derived from saturated fat. However, in 2015, the Dietary Guidelines Advisory Committee recommended doing away with an upper limit on dietary fat intake, and eliminating limits on cholesterol consumption, citing lack of evidence that these restrictions have ever been necessary for public health (Mozaffarian and Ludwig 2015).

Calcium and Vitamin D for Bone Health

Calcium is the most abundant mineral in the human body and the main constituent of bones and teeth. Its major food sources include dairy products, sardines with bones, fortified soymilk, turnip greens, kale, and fortified tofu. Vitamin D is a fat-soluble nutrient produced in the skin through exposure to the sun, and it facilitates the intestinal absorption of calcium. There are few natural food sources of vitamin D, but some include fatty fish, such as salmon, herring, and catfish, fish liver oil, and fortified milk. Achieving an adequate intake of calcium and sufficient blood levels of vitamin D during adolescence is crucial to physical growth and development. Because about half of total bone density is attained during adolescence, sufficient amounts of calcium and vitamin D during this stage in life are important for the accrual of dense bone mass, and the reduction of the lifetime risk of fractures and **osteoporosis**.

Starting at about age nine, children begin their critical bone-building years, and by the time they reach 18, they have developed almost all of their bone mass. Even after children and teens stop growing taller, they continue to make more bone than they lose. This mean their bones continue getting denser until they reach what is known as **peak bone mass**, the point when an individual has the greatest amount of bone that they will ever have. Peak bone mass is usually reached between the ages of 18 and 25. The more bone there is at the point of peak bone mass, the less likely a bone fracture will occur or that osteoporosis will develop later in life (National Osteoporosis Foundation n.d.). However, research studies show that many adolescents do not obtain adequate amounts of calcium or vitamin D (Harkness and Bonny 2005). The dietary reference intake (DRI) for calcium is 1,300 mg per day for both males and females ages 9 to 18. The DRI for vitamin D is 15 µg (600 IU) for both males and females ages 9 to 18.

Controllable Risk Factors for Osteoporosis

- Insufficient intake of calcium and vitamin D
- Insufficient intake of fruits and vegetables
- Excessive intake of protein, sodium and caffeine
- Sedentary lifestyle
- Smoking
- Excessive intake of alcohol
- Excessive weight loss

Source: National Osteoporosis Foundation (n.d.).

Iron

Iron is an essential component of hundreds of proteins and enzymes involved in many metabolic processes, including oxygen transport and energy metabolism. Adolescents have increased requirements for iron due to rapid growth, increased blood volume, and **cognitive** development. Adolescent girls in particular are at increased risk of iron deficiency due to inadequate dietary iron intake along with the iron loss that occurs with menstruation (Micronutrient Information Center 2012).

Iron deficiency during adolescence may impair immunity as well as growth and cognition (Micronutrient Information Center 2012). The adolescent's diet, therefore, must provide enough iron and other nutrients, such as vitamin C, that promote adequate iron **bioavailability** and utilization by the body. Many teenagers consume unbalanced diets with a lack of variety, which may limit their iron intake and hinder its bioavailability, leading to a possible deficiency (Mesias, Seiquer, and Seiquer 2013).

Alcohol, Smoking, and Drug Use

As children move from the early stages of adolescence into their middle and late teenage years, brain development is still in progress and continues into the early twenties. Research indicates that this extensive period of neurological development may explain the propensity adolescents have toward risk-taking behavior, and why they do not often fully recognize or anticipate the consequences of their actions. Some of these risky behaviors include alcohol consumption, smoking cigarettes, and experimenting with illicit drugs.

Alcohol

Many adolescents start to drink at very young ages. In 2003, the average age of first-time alcohol use was 14, compared to about 17½ in. 1965 (National Institute on Alcohol Abuse and Alcoholism 2006). By the time they are high-school seniors, almost 70 percent of teenagers will have tried alcohol (National Institute on Drug Abuse 2014).

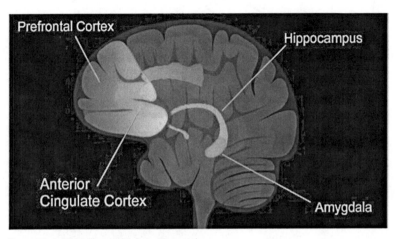

Source: National Institute of Medicine Image Library.

Such risk-taking behavior may have a biological basis. Researchers found that alcohol may impact teenagers differently compared to adults who drink. Adolescents appear to be more vulnerable to the negative effects of alcohol on the **hippocampus**—the part of the brain that regulates working memory and learning. As a result, heavy use of alcohol throughout the teenage years may hinder academic performance, as well as impair memory and attention span, even into one's early and mid-twenties (McNeely and Blanchard 2009).

If an adolescent begins drinking before age 15, they are four times more likely to become alcohol-dependent compared with those who do not start to drink until age 21. Teenagers also tend to be less sensitive to the sedative effects of alcohol, so they are able to stay awake longer with higher blood alcohol concentration compared with older drinkers, and therefore adolescents expose themselves to the possibility of greater cognitive impairment (McNeely and Blanchard 2009). This difference in sensitivity to alcohol may explain why many teenage drinkers can consume significantly larger amounts than do adults before experiencing the associated negative effects, such as drowsiness, lack of coordination, and symptoms of withdrawal; and it may also explain why there are high rates of **binge drinking** among young adults. According to a 2013 National Survey on Drug Use and Health (NSDUH), about 5.4 million teenagers aged 12 to 20 engaged in binge drinking (National Institute on Alcohol Abuse and Alcoholism n.d.).

Underage drinking is when anyone under the minimum legal drinking age of 21 drinks alcohol, and it is a widespread public health problem. Health risks of underage drinking include:

Death
As many as 4,358 people under age 21 die each year from alcohol-related car crashes, homicides, suicides, alcohol poisoning, and other injuries such as falls, burns, and drowning.

Serious injuries
More than 190,000 people under age 21 visited an emergency room for alcohol-related injuries in 2008.

Impaired judgment
Drinking can lead to poor judgment and decisions, which can then result in risky behavior like drinking and driving, sexual activity, or violence.

Increased risk for physical and sexual assault
Adolescents who drink are more likely to carry out or be the victim of a physical or sexual assault.

Brain development problems
Research shows that brain development continues well into a person's twenties. Alcohol can affect this development, and contribute to a range of memory and concentration problems (National Institute on Alcohol Abuse and Alcoholism n.d.).

Smoking

In a 2010 survey of American adolescents, about 2.6 million respondents aged 12 to 17 reported using a tobacco product in the prior month. In that same year, researchers found that almost 60 percent of new smokers were under the age of 18 (National Institute on Drug Abuse 2012).

Cigarettes contain **nicotine**, an oily liquid that is the main active constituent of tobacco, and acts as a **stimulant** in small doses. Smoking tobacco enables nicotine absorption through the lungs' air sacs, and regular smoking can result in cellular damage and cell loss throughout the brain at any age. In teenagers, such damage is worse in the hippocampus. In addition, compared to adults, adolescent smokers experience more episodes of depression and cardiac irregularities, and are more likely to become quickly dependent on nicotine (McNeely and Blanchard 2009).

Health risks associated with smoking during adolescence, include:

Respiratory effects
Reduced lung function and reduced rate of lung growth.
Shortness of breath
Teenage smokers suffer from shortness of breath almost three times as often as teens who don't smoke, and produce phlegm more than twice as often as teens who don't smoke.
Impaired physical fitness
Impacts performance and endurance.
Lung cancer
Smoking at an early age increases lifelong risk.
Addiction to nicotine
Nicotine is an addictive substance like alcohol and many illicit drugs.
Likelihood of continued smoking throughout adulthood
Many lifelong smokers began their habit during their teenage years.
Development of heart disease and stroke in adulthood
Studies have shown that early signs of these diseases can be found in adolescents who smoke.

Source: WHO (n.d.).

Drug Use

Illicit drug use during the adolescent years is an important predictor of the development of a substance abuse problem later in life. The majority of adults who suffer from drug addiction start using these substances before age 18. Twenty-five percent of those who begin abusing prescription drugs at age 13 or earlier, eventually develop a substance abuse problem at some point in their lives.

Unfortunately, teenagers are particularly vulnerable to drug addiction, because some parts of their brains remain immature, and are in a state of **neuroplasticity**—still capable of being altered by external experiences and influences. During childhood, the areas of the brain that process feelings of reward and pain, the very parts that lend themselves to drug use, happen to be the first to reach maturity. However, during adolescence, the **prefrontal cortex**, the very part of the brain that is responsible for evaluating situations, making good decisions, and controlling impulse, is still developing and is not mature until a person is in their mid-twenties (National Institute on Drug Abuse 2014).

At the same time, there are other factors that contribute to adolescent drug use, including drug availability within a neighborhood, school, or surrounding community; whether or not a teenager's friends are using drugs; and if the family environment involves physical or emotional abuse (McNeely and Blanchard 2009).

Many illicit drugs, such as cocaine, raise the body's level of **dopamine**, a brain chemical that influences the feelings of reward and pleasure. Drug use targets the brain's dopamine receptor neurons, damaging these cells and possibly affecting adolescent brain development for life in the areas of impulse control and the ability to experience reward (McNeely and Blanchard 2009).

The "high" produced by these drugs results from the inundation of the brain's reward circuits with far more dopamine than normal. This affect creates an especially strong desire to repeat the experience. Since an adolescent is already struggling with the need to balance impulse with self-control, it is more likely that they will take drugs again without adequate assessment of the consequences. With the repeated drug experiences, the brain circuitry increasingly reinforces the neural links between the feelings of pleasure and use of the drug.

Eventually, drug use may take on a level of importance in the adolescent's life out of proportion to other rewards, and compels them to reshuffle their priorities in unfortunate ways. Meanwhile, the brain's repeated exposure to the substance impacts its key areas necessary for judgment and self-control, further hindering the individual's ability to control or stop their drug use. Therefore, willpower alone is often not enough to overcome an addiction, because the drug use itself has compromised the very parts of the brain that makes it possible for a person to stop (National Institute on Drug Abuse 2014).

A repeated pattern of drug use poses serious social and health risks, including

- Academic failure,
- Social problems with family and peers,
- Loss of interest in normal healthy activities,
- Impaired memory,
- Exposure to infectious diseases, such as HIV or hepatitis C, through risky sexual behavior or sharing contaminated injection equipment,
- Mental health problems, and
- Death due to overdose.

Source: National Institute on Drug Abuse (2014).

Adolescent Obesity

Child and adolescent obesity is a serious public health problem in the United States. It has more than doubled in children and quadrupled in adolescents in the past 30 years. In 2012, more than one-third of children

1 get over the idea of magic foods
There are no magic foods to eat for good health. Teen guys need to eat foods such as vegetables, fruits, whole grains, protein foods, and fat-free or low-fat dairy foods. Choose protein foods like unsalted nuts, beans, lean meats, and fish. SuperTracker.usda.gov will show if you are getting the nutrients you need for growth.

2 always hungry?
Whole grains that provide fiber can give you a feeling of fullness and provide key nutrients. Choose half your grains as whole grains. Eat whole-wheat breads, pasta, and brown rice instead of white bread, rice, or other refined grains. Also, choose vegetables and fruits when you need to "fill-up."

3 keep water handy
Water is a better option than many other drink choices. Keep a water bottle in your backpack and at your desk to satisfy your thirst. Skip soda, fruit drinks, and energy and sports drinks. They are sugar-sweetened and have few nutrients.

4 make a list of favorite foods
Like green apples more than red apples? Ask your

6 skip foods that can add unwanted pounds
Cut back on calories by limiting fatty meats like ribs, bacon, and hot dogs. Some foods are just occasional treats like pizza, cakes, cookies, candies, and ice cream. Check out the calorie content of sugary drinks by reading the Nutrition Facts label. Many 12-ounce sodas contain 10 teaspoons of sugar.

7 learn how much food you need
Teen guys may need more food than most adults, teen girls, and little kids. Go to www.SuperTracker.usda.gov. It shows how much food you need based on your age, height, weight, and activity level. It also tracks progress towards fitness goals. **SuperTracker**

8 check Nutrition Facts labels
To grow, your body needs vitamins and minerals. Calcium and vitamin D are especially important for your growing bones. Read Nutrition Facts labels for calcium. Dairy foods provide the minerals your bones need to grow.

9 strengthen your muscles
Work on strengthening and aerobic

Source: www.choosemyplate.gov/sites/default/files/tentips/DGTipsheet34ChooseTheFoodsYouNeedToGrow.pdf

1 build strong bones
A good diet and regular physical activity can build strong bones throughout your life. Choose fat-free or low-fat milk, cheeses, and yogurt to get the vitamin D and calcium your growing bones need. Strengthen your bones three times a week doing activities such as running, gymnastics, and skating.

2 cut back on sweets
Cut back on sugary drinks. Many 12-ounce cans of soda have 10 teaspoons of sugar in them. Drink water when you are thirsty. Sipping water and cutting back on cakes, candies, and sweets helps to maintain a healthy weight.

3 power up with whole grain
Fuel your body with nutrient-packed whole-grain foods. Make sure that at least half your grain foods are whole grains such as brown rice, whole-wheat breads, and popcorn.

4 choose vegetables rich in color

6 be a healthy role model
Encourage your friends to practice healthier habits. Share what you do to work through challenges. Keep your computer and TV time to less than 2 hours a day (unless it's school work).

7 try something new
Keep healthy eating fun by picking out new foods you've never tried before like lentils, mango, quinoa, or kale.

8 make moving part of every event
Being active makes everyone feel good. Aim for 60 minutes of physical activity each day. Move your body often. Dancing, playing active games, walking to school with friends, swimming, and biking are only a few fun ways to be active. Also, try activities that target the muscles in your arms and legs.

9 include all food groups daily
Use MyPlate as your guide to include all food groups each day. Learn more at www.ChooseMyPlate.gov.

Source: www.choosemyplate.gov/sites/default/files/tentips/DGTipsheet36EatSmartAndBeActiveAsYouGrow.pdf

and adolescents were overweight or obese. Approximately 17 percent of children and adolescents aged 2 to 19 (12.7 million people) years are obese, a prevalence that has remained steady since 2003. From 1980 to 2012, the percentage of adolescents aged 12 to 19 who were classified as obese increased from 5 to 21 percent (Centers for Disease Control and Prevention 2015a).

Childhood obesity is also more common among certain racial and ethnic groups. In 2011 to 2012, the prevalence among children and adolescents was higher among Hispanics (22.4 percent) and non-Hispanic blacks (20.2 percent) than among non-Hispanic whites (14.1 percent). The prevalence of obesity was lower in non-Hispanic Asian youth (8.6 percent) than in youth who were non-Hispanic white, non-Hispanic black or Hispanic (Centers for Disease Control and Prevention 2015a).

Obesity is defined as having a body mass index (BMI) at or above the 95th percentile for age and gender on the growth charts developed by the Centers for Disease Control and Prevention (CDC). A predisposition to obesity can be inherited. However, genetic factors do not explain the dramatic increase in obesity over the last three decades (McNeely and Blanchard 2009). The current prevalence of child and adolescent obesity stems from a complex interconnection of factors that include genetic predisposition, sedentary lifestyle, and environmental influence.

Some of the factors that contribute to adolescent obesity are the following:

- The disproportionate sale of high-fat, high-calorie foods and sugary drinks in schools compared with healthier choices.
- Limited access to healthier food options in low-income communities.
- Sedentary habits of adolescents due to an excessive amount of screen time.
- Reduced number of school physical education programs.
- Excessive media advertising of unhealthy products targets at children and teenagers.
- Oversized portions that provide more calories than adolescents need.
- Genetic factors. A child under 10 years of age with obese parents faces double the risk of becoming an obese adult.
- Fast food consumption. On average, adolescents eat at fast food restaurants twice a week.

Source: OWH (2012).

Obesity and Health Risks

Obesity increases the risk for various chronic diseases, as well as psychological issues for children and teenagers that often continue into adulthood. Obese youth are more likely to have risk factors for cardiovascular disease, such as high cholesterol or high blood pressure. In a population-based study of 5- to 17-year-olds, 70 percent of obese youth had at least one risk factor for cardiovascular disease. Obese adolescents are more likely to have prediabetes, a condition in which blood glucose levels indicate a high risk for development of diabetes. Children and adolescents who are obese are at greater risk for bone and joint problems, **sleep apnea**, and social and psychological issues, such as **stigmatization** and low self-esteem.

The majority of overweight teenagers become obese adults, since eating patterns established in childhood often extend into later life, and they are therefore more at risk for adult health problems, such as heart disease, type 2 diabetes, stroke, several types of cancer, and **osteoarthritis** (Centers for Disease Control and Prevention 2015b).

Obesity Treatment and Interventions

Strategies involving prevention and early intervention are central to reversing the obesity epidemic among American youth. These efforts would have to draw from multiple disciplines, including use of professionals in the fields of medicine, psychology, nutrition, and exercise physiology—working together to facilitate family-centered behavior change. Since family habits and cultural traditions heavily influence adolescent eating behavior, any behavioral treatment and counseling approach should be implemented with these considerations in mind to achieve small, gradual goals in food habits and physical activity. Any program of intervention should also emphasize gradual weight loss rather than a quick return to normal BMI to ensure continued normal growth and development. However, severe obesity cases may require further assessment for surgical and pharmacological approaches if other treatments fail (Gurnani, Birken, and Hamilton 2015).

The Athletic Teen

For some adolescents, sports participation is a big part of their lives, either recreationally or for competition. The nutrient requirements to support athletic activity are, by and large, the same that define overall healthy eating and optimum nourishment. Teenagers who eat healthy, balanced meals and snacks will likely obtain all the nutrients they need to perform well in sports. However, an athletic teenager will have higher energy and fluid requirements compared with their more sedentary peers.

Energy

Balancing energy intake with energy expenditure is crucial to preventing too little or too much calorie consumption. Energy deficits can lead to shortness of stature, a delay in the onset of puberty, menstrual dysfunction, loss of muscle mass, and increased likelihood of fatigue, injury, or illness. However, excess energy intake can result in overweight and obesity, even for athletes (Purcell, Canadian Paediatric Society, and Paediatric Sports and Exercise Medicine Section 2013).

Fluids

Adolescent athletes need to drink adequate amounts of fluids to prevent dehydration, which can in turn impact strength, energy, and coordination, and also lead to heat-related illness. Fluids help regulate body temperature and replace sweat losses during exercise. Proper hydration requires fluid intake before, during, and after exercise, and self-assessment of thirst is not a reliable method for determining hydration status. Before activity, athletes should consume 16 to 24 oz of water two to three hours before an event. During an activity, athletes should consume 4 to 6 oz of fluid every 15 to 20 minutes. For events lasting less than one hour, water is sufficient. For events lasting longer than 60 minutes or taking place in hot, humid weather, sports drinks containing carbohydrates and **electrolytes**, such as **sodium** and **potassium**, which athletes lose in sweat, are a good option. For nonathletes, routine consumption of carbohydrate-containing sports drinks can result in excessive calorie intake (Purcell 2013).

Macronutrients

Carbohydrates are the most important fuel source for athletes at any age, because they provide a quick source of glucose, which is used for immediate and sustained energy. Glucose is stored in the form of glycogen in the muscles and liver. Muscle glycogen is the most readily available source of energy for working muscles, and it can be released more rapidly than other energy sources. Therefore, carbohydrates should comprise 45 to 65 percent of total caloric intake in an athletic teenager's diet (Purcell, Canadian Paediatric Society, and Paediatric Sports and Exercise Medicine Section 2013).

For mild exercise of short duration, protein does not serve as a primary fuel source. However, as the duration of exercise increases, protein can help maintain blood glucose levels through a process known as **gluconeogenesis**. Protein should comprise approximately 10 to 30 percent of total energy intake (Purcell, Canadian Paediatric Society, and Paediatric Sports and Exercise Medicine Section 2013).

Fat is necessary to absorb fat-soluble vitamins, provide essential fatty acids, protect vital organs, and provide insulation. It is a calorie-dense source of energy. Fats should comprise 25 to 35 percent of total energy in the athlete's diet.

Micronutrients

Although there are many vitamins and minerals required for good health, young athletes should pay special attention to consuming proper amounts of calcium, vitamin D, and iron (Purcell, Canadian Paediatric Society, and Paediatric Sports and Exercise Medicine Section 2013).

Calcium is important for bone health, normal enzyme activity, and muscle contraction. Vitamin D is also necessary for bone health and is involved in the absorption and regulation of calcium. Athletes who live in northern latitudes or who predominantly train indoors are likely to be vitamin D deficient. Iron is important for oxygen delivery to body tissues. During adolescence, more iron is required to support growth as well as the increases in blood volume and lean muscle mass. In athletes, iron depletion is common because of unbalanced eating habits or because of increased iron losses in menstrual blood. Therefore, athletes, particularly, female athletes, and vegetarians should be screened periodically for iron status (Purcell, Canadian Paediatric Society, and Paediatric Sports and Exercise Medicine Section 2013).

Body Image

Adolescence is a critical period for establishing a healthy **body image**, which can be challenging for most teenagers given the type and extent of the developmental transitions that occur. The changes that unfold during puberty are among the most rapid and diverse in human development, including changes in weight, height, body shape, body composition, as well as primary and secondary sex characteristics. These transformative steps coincide with increased exposure to media and societal messages on idealized versions of physical beauty, which in turn influence eating habits and attitudes toward food (Voelker, Reel, and Greenleaf 2015).

Body image is a complex mental picture of how individuals perceive, think, feel, and act toward their bodies, and can be viewed as lying on a continuum from healthy body perception to unhealthy body perception. Research evidence indicates that unhealthy body image is associated with obesity and physical inactivity and plays a highly influential role in the development of eating disorders during adolescence (Voelker, Reel, and Greenleaf 2015).

Disordered Eating versus Eating Disorder

Disordered eating describes a variety of abnormal eating behaviors that observed on their own are not individually classified as an *eating disorder*, which is a distinct psychological illness. Rather, disordered eating includes behaviors that are known common features of eating disorders, such as chronic restrained eating, compulsive eating, binge eating, and self-induced vomiting. Certain factors among adolescents tend to be associated with disordered eating, including BMI, negative mood, level of self-esteem, emphasis on perfectionism, drug use, perceived pressure to lose weight, and participation in sports and other activities, such as dance, that emphasize physical leanness.

An eating disorder is a mental disorder defined by abnormal eating habits that negatively impact a person's physical or mental health. The most commonly known eating disorders include the following:

Binge Eating Disorder
Eating an inordinate amount of food in a short period of time without subsequent purging episodes.

Anorexia Nervosa
Characterized by tremendous fear and anxiety over gaining weight, combined with a strong desire to be thin and enormous food restriction. Many people with anorexia see themselves as overweight. If asked, they usually deny they have a problem. They weigh themselves frequently, eat only small amounts of certain foods. Many anorexics will exercise excessively, force themselves to vomit, or use laxatives to produce weight loss. Complications may include osteoporosis, infertility, and heart damage.

Bulimia Nervosa
Characterized by binge eating followed by purging, which refers to attempts to rid oneself of the food consumed. This may be done by vomiting or taking a **laxative**. Other efforts to lose weight may include use of a **diuretic** or a stimulant, fasting, or excessive exercise.

Eating disorders are more likely to occur during and shortly after puberty. Ninety-five percent of those who have an eating disorder are between the ages of 12 and 25; and females are much more likely than males to develop the condition. An estimated 85 to 95 percent of eating disorder sufferers are girls or women; and eating disorders have the highest death rate of any mental illness. Twenty percent of people suffering from anorexia die prematurely from complications related to the disease, including those who die from suicide or heart problems (National Association of Anorexia Nervosa and Associated Disorders n.d.).

As health and medical experts continue to struggle to figure out why a disproportionate number of young females develop eating disorders, the prevailing theories factor in the increased adipose tissue that develops in girls, the hormonal changes involved in puberty, and societal pressure to conform to cultural ideals of feminine beauty.

In general, boys report lower levels of body dissatisfaction and exhibit fewer disordered eating behaviors compared to girls. However, rather than striving for thinness, boys are more likely than girls to be concerned with muscularity. Data from the United States, Canada, and Australia indicate that underweight or obese adolescent males are more likely than healthy weight males to be dissatisfied with their bodies. Consequently, some boys pursue muscularity and low body fat percentage through overeating and using **anabolic steroids** (Calzo et al. 2015).

Key Terms

Anabolic Steroids
A synthetically produced hormone that is sometimes used illegally by athletes to help them increase the size and strength of their muscles, and improve endurance.

Binge Drinking
The practice of consuming large quantities of alcohol in a single session (typically two hours), and defined as five or more drinks at one time.

Bioavailability
The extent to which a nutrient can be used by the body.

Body Image
The subjective mental image of one's own body.

Cognitive
Related to the mental processes of perception, memory, judgment, thinking, and reasoning.

Diuretic
A substance that increases the flow of urine.

Dopamine
A brain chemical that plays a role in cognition, motivation, attention, mood, sleep, voluntary movement, learning, and working memory.

Electrolytes
Salts and minerals that can conduct electrical impulses in the body. They control the body's fluid balance and are important in muscle contraction, energy production, and major biochemical reactions.

Gluconeogenesis
The synthesis of glucose by the liver from noncarbohydrate sources through the conversion of certain amino acids, pyruvate, lactate, or glycerol.

Hippocampus
A small, curved formation in the brain that plays an important role in storing memories, connecting them with emotions, and learning.

Laxative
A food or drug that stimulates evacuation of the bowels. Used to alleviate constipation.

Neurological
The science of the nerves and the nervous system, especially of the diseases affecting them.

Neuroplasticity
The process in which the brain reorganizes itself by forming new neural connections throughout life. It allows the nerve cells in the brain

to compensate for injury and disease and to adjust their activities in response to new situations or to changes in the environment.

Nicotine
A chemical compound that is present in tobacco leaves. When tobacco is smoked, nicotine is absorbed through the wall lining of the small air sacs in the lungs. When sniffed or chewed, it is absorbed through the mucous membranes of the nose or mouth.

Osteoarthritis
A degenerative joint disease; a type of arthritis that develops when flexible tissue at the end of bones wears down.

Osteoporosis
Literally "porous bone." A medical condition in which the bones become increasingly porous, brittle, and vulnerable to fractures due to the depletion of calcium and protein in the skeletal system.

Peak Bone Mass
The largest amount of bone tissue a person will ever have throughout their life.

Potassium
The body's major positively charged electrolyte (ion) inside the cells. Important for regulating heart beat and muscle function.

Prefrontal Cortex
The part of the brain located just behind the forehead, and is responsible for regulating higher-level thinking skills and behavior. This includes decision making between right and wrong, and predicting the consequences of actions or events.

Secondary Sexual Characteristics
Any of a number of physical characteristics developing at puberty, such as the appearance of the breasts, beard, enlarged muscles, distribution of fat tissue, or change in voice pitch that is specific to each sex, but not essential to reproduction.

Sleep Apnea

A sleep disorder in which there are intermittent pauses in breathing during sleep and often results in sleepiness during the day. Excess weight and smoking are among the risk factors.

Sodium

The body's major positively charged electrolyte (ion) outside the cells. Obtained primarily through the consumption of sodium chloride (table salt) in the diet. Important for fluid balance.

Stigmatization

The circumstance of being labeled or described as deserving of public disapproval.

Stimulant

A substance that increases alertness and energy; elevates blood pressure, heart rate, and respiration; often touted as a weight loss aid.

References

Calzo, J.P., K.E. Masyn, H.L. Corliss, E.A. Scherer, A.E. Field, and S.B. Austin. 2015. "Patterns of Body Image Concerns and Disordered Weight- and Shape-Related Behaviors in Heterosexual and Sexual Minority Adolescent Males." *Developmental Psychology* 51, no. 9, pp. 1216–25.

Centers for Disease Control and Prevention. June 19, 2015a. "Childhood Obesity Facts." www.cdc.gov/obesity/data/childhood.html (accessed November 4, 2015).

Centers for Disease Control and Prevention. August 27, 2015b. "Health Effects of Childhood Obesity." www.cdc.gov/healthyschools/obesity/facts.htm (accessed November 4, 2015).

Gurnani, M., C. Birken, and J. Hamilton. August 2015. "Childhood Obesity: Causes, Consequences and Management." *Pediatric Clinics of North America* 62, no. 4, pp. 821–40.

Harkness, L.S., and A.E. Bonny. November 2005. "Calcium and Vitamin D Status in the Adolescent: Key Roles for Bone, Body Weight, Glucose Tolerance, and Estrogen Biosynthesis." *Journal of Pediatric and Adolescent Gynecology* 18, no. 5, pp. 305–11.

McNeely, C., and J. Blanchard. 2010. *The Teen Years Explained: A Guide to Healthy Adolescent Development.* Baltimore, MD: The Center for Adolescent Health at Johns Hopkins Bloomberg School of Public Health.

Mesias, M., I. Seiquer, and M.P. Seiquer. 2013. "Iron Nutrition in Adolescence." *Critical Reviews in Food Science and Nutrition* 53, no. 11, pp. 1226–37.

Micronutrient Information Center. July 2012. Linus Pauling Institute. Oregon State University. www.lpi.oregonstate.edu/mic/life-stages/adolescents (accessed November 1, 2015).

Mozaffarian, D., and D.S. Ludwig. June 2015. "The 2015 US Dietary Guidelines. Lifting the Ban on Total Dietary Fat." *Journal of the American Medical Association* 313, no. 24, pp. 2421–22.

National Association of Anorexia Nervosa and Associated Disorders. n.d. "Eating Disorders Statistics." www.anad.org/get-information/about-eating-disorders/eating-disorders-statistics/ (accessed November 13, 2015).

National Institute on Alcohol Abuse and Alcoholism. January 2006. "Underage Drinking - Why Do Adolescents Drink, What Are the Risks, and How Can Underage Drinking Be Prevented?" http://pubs.niaaa.nih.gov/publications/AA67/AA67.htm (accessed November 1, 2015).

National Institute on Alcohol Abuse and Alcoholism. n.d. "Underage Drinking." www.niaaa.nih.gov/alcohol-health/special-populations-co-occurring-disorders/underage-drinking (accessed November 1, 2015).

National Institute on Drug Abuse. January 2014. "Principles of Adolescent Substance Use Disorder Treatment: A Research Based Guide." www.drugabuse.gov/publications/principles-adolescent-substance-use-disorder-treatment-research-based-guide/introduction (accessed November 2, 2015).

National Institute on Drug Abuse. July 2012. "Smoking and Adolesence." www.drugabuse.gov/publications/research-reports/tobacco/smoking-adolescence (accessed November 2, 2015).

National Osteoporosis Foundation. n.d. "Bone Basics." www.nof.org/learn/bonebasics (accessed October 7, 2015).

OWH (Office of Women's Health). September 2012. "Bodyworks: A Toolkit for Healthy Teens & Strong Families (Body Basics)." U.S. Department of Health and Human Services. www.womenshealth.gov/bodyworks/current-trainers/bodyworks-toolkit/toolkit.parents.pdf

Purcell, L.K., Canadian Paediatric Society, and Paediatric Sports and Exercise Medicine Section. April 2013. "Sport Nutrition for Young Athletes." *Paediatric Child Health* 18, no. 4, pp. 200–5.

Voelker, D.K., J.J. Reel, and C. Greenleaf. 2015. "Weight Status and Body Image Perceptions in Adolescents: Current Perspectives." *Adolescent Health, Medicine and Therapeutics* 6, pp. 149–58.

WHO (World Health Organization). n.d. "Health Effects of Smoking Among Young People." www.who.int/tobacco/research/youth/health_effects/en/ (accessed November 2, 2015).

CHAPTER 6

The Older Adult

Introduction

To date, the person who reached the oldest verifiable age in history was Jeanne Calment, a French woman. Born in 1875, she lived to be 122 years old and died in 1997.

While the average human **life span** has yet to reach such a staggering number, the percentage of people from around the world who are centenarians (aged 100 years or more) has been steadily increasing for the past 50 years. In 2011, the number of centenarians worldwide numbered 317,000 and is expected to increase to 3,224,000 by the year 2050, and to reach 17,795,000 by the end of the century (Evans et al. 2014).

Scientific research will likely never uncover a method to reverse aging, but ongoing studies may reveal ways to improve the quality of life of people as they age, mainly through examining how factors such as genes, environment, and behavioral influences, including diet, impact the human life span (National Institute on Aging 2011).

This final chapter addresses the changing nutritional needs of the older adult, which is defined as age 65 and older, and how meeting these important physiological requirements through healthy diet and exercise are vital to enjoying better quality years, and managing chronic diseases that tend to be more common in this age group.

Changing Demographics

In the United States, older adults are among the fastest growing age groups ("Healthy People 2020 Older Adults" n.d.). Since 1900, the percentage of Americans age 65 and older has more than tripled—from 4.1 to 13.1 percent of the population in 2010 (Bernstein and Munoz 2012). As of 2013, the number of people in the United States that were age 65 and

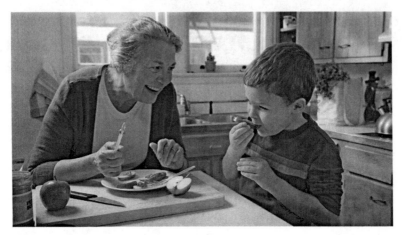

Source: https://snaped.fns.usda.gov/older-woman-and-young-boy-prepare-healthy-snack

older reached 44.7 million, and accounted for 14.1 percent of the total population (U.S. Census Bureau, Population Estimates 2013). By 2030, there will be about 72.1 million older adults, representing 19.3 percent of the population (Bernstein and Munoz 2012). That number is expected to increase to 98.2 million people by 2060—a group that would comprise nearly 25 percent of U.S. residents. In addition, 19.7 million of them would be age 85 or older (U.S. Census Bureau, Population Estimates 2014).

Currently, among Americans who are age 65 and older, the leading causes of death include heart disease, cancer, lower respiratory disease, stroke, Alzheimer's disease, and diabetes mellitus (Centers for Disease Control and Prevention 2014a). Many of these conditions are **chronic diseases**, and to a significant extent, nutrition status influences the trajectory and outcome of these health problems.

In addition, about one-fifth of people age 70 and older have visual impairments, placing them at greater risk of falls and other injury causes; and a third of older adults are hearing impaired. By 2030, more than 37 million older adults will face more than one chronic condition, many of which lead to disabilities, hospitalizations, loss of independence, and the need for nursing home care ("Healthy People 2020 Older Adults" n.d.).

Some of these illnesses overlap and result in complex conditions that require professional expertise to handle. Though most U.S. health care providers do receive some level of training related to health and aging, unfortunately, the percentage of those who actually specialize in this area is still small. Therefore, more trained specialists are needed to meet the needs of the country's aging population, and one of the new goals included in Healthy People 2020 is to increase the proportion of the health care workforce that obtains some type of **geriatric** certification in their area of practice. This call for more targeted expertise in treating the aging is aimed at many different health professionals, including physicians, psychiatrists, registered nurses, dentists, physical therapists, and registered dietitians ("Healthy People 2020 Older Adults" n.d.).

Nutrition and Health Promotion

While aging is obviously unavoidable, the physical frailties typically associated with it are not necessarily inevitable. Many people over 65 live relatively healthy and highly functioning lives. Approximately one-third of older adults are "aging successfully," and more than 39 percent of all noninstitutionalized people age 65 years and older are in excellent health (Bernstein and Munoz 2012).

Although there are many contributing factors to **successful aging**, good nutrition is one of the major determinants. Access to and the availability of wholesome and nutritious food is not only critical to meeting physiologic needs, but they also promote sustainably good physical and

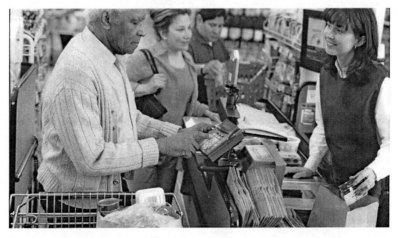

Source: https://snaped.fns.usda.gov/older-adult-man-purchasing-groceries-snap-benefits

psychological health, functionality, and the prevention of chronic diseases and their associated complications (Bernstein and Munoz 2012).

The exact nutrition needs of an older adult at any age vary because of the many differences in health status within this population. While the physiologic changes that occur with aging affect nutrient needs, actual nutrient requirements differ based on a person's individual circumstances, and not necessarily on chronological age. Generally, in older adults, a diet consistent with current federal guidelines, including relatively high amounts of vegetables, fruits, whole grains, poultry, fish, and low-fat dairy products has been associated with optimal nutritional status and reduced **mortality** (Bernstein and Munoz 2012).

The *MyPlate for Older Adults* visual guide may be a helpful reference guide, as it is designed to emphasize nutrition recommendations particularly important throughout the advancing years, such as adequate fluid intake; affordable and readily available foods; and physical activity. To download a pdf, go to: www.nia.nih.gov/sites/all/themes/woyp/pdf/tipsheets-myplate.pdf

MyPlate for Older Adults provides examples of foods that contain high levels of vitamins and minerals per serving and are consistent with the federal government's *2010 Dietary Guidelines for Americans*, which recommend limiting foods high in trans and saturated fats, salt and added sugars, and emphasize whole grains. The design features different forms of vegetables and fruits that are convenient, affordable, and readily available and icons that represent regular physical activity and highlight adequate fluid intake, both of particular concern for older adults. It offers several examples of liquids such as water, tea, coffee, and soup to address the common, age-related decline in thirst that can put older adults at risk for dehydration.

The physical activity icons depict common activities that include daily errands and household chores. Although some of those chores do not take the place of more formalized exercise routines involving cardiovascular exercises, they serve as a reminder of the many options for regular physical activity. The Dietary Guidelines also recommend limiting sodium intake to less than 1,500 mg per day, so spices and low-sodium options are suggested as alternatives.

Energy Needs

Calorie needs decline with age due to a decrease in metabolism and physical activity; however, nutritional requirements remain the same or in some cases increase. Therefore, meeting micronutrient and macronutrient needs with fewer calories can be challenging, leaving older adults more vulnerable to deficiencies.

Energy expenditure declines by about 15 percent between ages 30 and 80 (Bernstein and Munoz 2012). Based on broad federal guidelines, the estimated energy requirements for adults older than 50 is 2,400 calories per day. However, calorie level is highly variable, and should be individualized based on age, activity level, and gender. More specifically

A woman over age 50 should consume about
1,600 calories per day if physical activity is low.
1,800 calories per day if moderately active.
2,000 to 2,200 calories per day if highly active.

A man over age 50 should consume about
2,000 to 2,200 calories per day if physical activity is low.
2,200 to 2,400 calories per day if moderately active.
2,400 to 2,800 calories per day if highly active.

Activity levels
Low—activities associated with typical day-to-day life.
Moderate—the equivalent of walking 1.5 to 3 miles a day at 3 to 4 miles per hour.
High—the equivalent of walking more than 3 miles a day at 3 to 4 miles per hour.

Source: National Institutes of Health (2014).

Table 6.1 is a summary of information from several *Daily Food Plans* based on age and calorie level from the U.S. Department of Agriculture's (USDA) *Choose My Plate* website. To access individual food plans go to: www.choosemyplate.gov/tools-daily-food-plans.

Table 6.1 Summary of food groups and daily serving recommendations based on calorie level

Age (years)	Calorie level	Grains	Vegetables	Fruits	Dairy	Protein
18+	1,600	5 oz	2 cups	1½ cups	3 cups	5 oz
18+	1,800	6 oz	2½ cups	1½ cups	3 cups	5 oz
18+	2,000	6 oz	2½ cups	2 cups	3 cups	5½ oz
18+	2,200	7 oz	3 cups	2 cups	3 cups	6 oz
18+	2,400	8 oz	3 cups	2 cups	3 cups	6½ oz
18+	2,600	9 oz	3½	2 cups	3 cups	6½ oz

What Is a Serving

Grains: a 1-oz serving equivalent is one slice of bread; one ounce of ready-to-eat cereal; ½ cup of cooked rice, pasta, or cereal.

Vegetables: a serving is equivalent to one cup of raw or cooked vegetables; two cups of leafy salad greens; and one cup of 100 percent vegetable juice.

Fruits: a serving is equivalent to one cup of raw or cooked fruit, ½ cup of dried fruit, and one cup of 100 percent fruit juice.

Dairy: one serving is equivalent to one cup of milk, yogurt, or fortified soy beverage, 1½ oz of natural cheese, and 2 oz of processed cheese.

Protein Foods: one serving is equivalent to 1 oz of lean meat, poultry, or seafood; one egg; one tablespoon of peanut butter, ¼ cup of cooked beans or peas; ½ oz of nuts or seeds.

Fluid

The adequate intake (AI) of 2.7 L per day (about 11 cups) of water from food and beverages is an amount intended to replace normal daily losses and prevent dehydration, which is a major problem in older adults, especially those older than 85. The decreased ability of the kidneys to concentrate urine, a diminished thirst sensation, declining mental status, and side effects of medications are among the major risk factors for dehydration in older adults. In addition, fear of **incontinence** may discourage some people from consuming enough fluids. While the recommended AI serves as a general guideline, a more individualized recommendation calls for taking in 1 milliliter (mL) of fluid for every calorie consumed. Dehydration can result in constipation, **fecal impaction**, cognitive impairment, functional decline, and even death (Bernstein and Munoz 2012).

Carbohydrate

The recommended intake for carbohydrate is the same throughout adulthood, which is between 45 and 65 percent of total calories. Following the USDA's *Choose My Plate* recommendations ensures that the quantity and quality of carbohydrate is sufficient, and includes adequate amounts of fiber. To meet carbohydrate and fiber recommendations, older adults should choose a variety of fruits, vegetables, and sources of whole grains.

However, older adults who are frail, and those who have a poor appetite should be evaluated carefully, so that a diet high in fiber does not lead to excess feelings of fullness. Quick satiety could decrease daily food consumption, hinder adequate nutrient intake, and contribute to unintentional weight loss. Moreover, any recommendations for dietary fiber intake must take fluid needs into account as well, since water needs increase with higher fiber consumption (Bernstein and Munoz 2012).

Protein

Insufficient resources, reduced appetite, and physical limitations can make adequate consumption of high-quality protein sources difficult for older adults to achieve on a regular basis. A decrease in total body protein with advancing age contributes to increased frailty, impaired wound healing, and diminished immune function. Studies suggest that the requirement for dietary protein in older adults is the same as that for healthy younger adults, and that the Recommended Dietary Allowance (RDA) of 0.8 g of protein per kg of body weight per day is adequate to meet minimum dietary needs (Bernstein and Munoz 2012).

However, some experts believe that a higher amount of daily protein would be beneficial. Although the role of dietary protein in the prevention of muscle atrophy remains unclear, a protein intake moderately greater than the RDA may help preserve lean body mass. A daily intake of 1.0 to 1.6 g per kg is considered safe for healthy older adults. For both the young and old, studies suggest that the most protein from a single meal that the body can use for building muscle is approximately 30 g. Therefore, some experts recommend that older adults aim to consume between 25 and 30 g high-quality protein at each meal (Bernstein and Munoz 2012). "High quality" refers to protein sources that contain all nine essential amino acids, such as meat, poultry, and eggs; or plant-based complementary sources, such as rice and beans; pasta and vegetables; bread and nut butters.

Fats

As discussed in previous chapters, dietary fats are essential to good health by contributing to normal signal transmission between cells, comprising the structure of cellular membranes, protecting the body's organs, and facilitating the absorption of the fat-soluble vitamins.

To date, recommendations suggest that all adults consume no more than 25 to 35 percent of calories from fat, with up to 10 percent derived from saturated fat. However, in 2015, the Dietary Guidelines Advisory Committee recommended doing away with an upper limit on dietary fat intake, and eliminating limits on cholesterol consumption, citing lack of evidence that these restrictions confer any health benefits (Mozaffarian and Ludwig 2015).

One area of particular relevance for older adults are the recent studies of the link between essential fatty acids and cognitive function. Research shows promising evidence that omega-3 fatty acid consumption, primarily from fish oil, may play a role in the prevention or delay in progression of Alzheimer's disease, though far more research is needed to draw any firm conclusions (Thomas et al. 2015).

Vitamin B12

An estimated 6 to 15 percent of older adults have a vitamin B12 deficiency (Bernstein and Munoz 2012), a nutrient that is naturally found only in animal products; certain types of edible algae and fermented foods; and fortified grains or other fortified products. Vitamin B12 is important for the health of nerve and red blood cells, and levels are commonly low in older adults as a result of impaired absorption due to **pernicious anemia**, a condition that impairs production of **intrinsic factor**. Another cause of deficiency can be **atrophic gastritis**, and in some cases poor diet. Deficiency symptoms include **megaloblastic anemia**, which causes weakness and fatigue, and severe deficiency may result in neurological complications, such as numbness and tingling in the hands and feet, memory problems, poor balance, and depression. Vitamin B12 deficiency is normally treated with an intramuscular injection of the nutrient, as well as high-dose dietary supplements.

Vitamin D and Calcium

In later adulthood, adequate vitamin D and calcium play a crucial role in the prevention and delay of progression of osteoporosis. Both nutrients have also been studied for their role in reducing the risk of cancer, heart disease, diabetes, and immunity-related conditions. The current dietary reference intakes (DRIs) are based on evidence that supports calcium and vitamin D's importance to bone health, but not for other medical issues. The Institute of Medicine (IOM) has cautioned that too much of these nutrients in supplement form may be harmful according to some studies (Bernstein and Munoz 2012).

Current recommendations include consuming as much as the DRI for calcium and vitamin D as possible through food, and then using a dietary supplement to close any gaps in intake. The DRI for adults older than 50 is 1,200 mg of calcium per day, and 15 µg (600 IU) of vitamin D per day for adults ages 51 to 70; and 20 µg (800 IU) of vitamin D per day for adults older than 70.

Understanding Longevity

As a greater number of adults experience increasing **longevity**, researchers are working to understand why some people experience their older years relatively free of disease and major health problems, while others face extreme challenges. Studies of people with exceptional longevity are helping to explain these differences in declining health and increased **morbidity** with old age and why some people have the ability to resist disease better than others. For example, do major health problems start around the same age in all people and then worsen through the many added years of a long life, or is there a delay in the onset of disease to begin with in those who live to be 100? (National Institute on Aging 2011).

Observational studies have indicated that the average centenarian seems to be in better health than the average 80-year-old. To understand the genetic and lifestyle factors that may explain these observations, investigators have looked to an area of science known as **epigenetics** to better understand longevity, and how to delay or prevent diseases and disabilities commonly associated with aging (National Institute on Aging 2011).

Research into epigenetics explores to what extent the environment affects how genes function and influences health and aging. Epigenetics is a process that refers to external chemical modifications to DNA that do not change its sequence. Instead, these modifications or "marks" on DNA influence whether or not certain genes are activated (gene expression) or suppressed. Collectively, these marks on DNA are known as the **epigenome**, which changes the way cells use DNA instructions.

Lifestyle and environmental factors, such as smoking, diet, medication, and pollutants may alter some of the marks on DNA, which

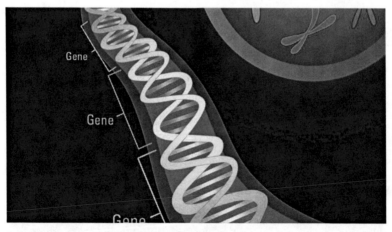

Source: National Institute of Medicine Image Library.

in turn causes a modification of gene activity. Most epigenetic changes are thought to be harmless, but researchers believe that some could trigger diseases such as cancer or diabetes, or exacerbate an already existing condition (National Institute on Aging 2011).

While scientists are still far away from making definitive dietary recommendations that address issues related to aging and disease, further study of nutrition and epigenetics may pave the way for a better quality of life with less illness and disability in the aging population.

The Impact of Chronic Disease

It is well established that some combination of genetic vulnerability and environmental factors is responsible for the rising prevalence of chronic disease in the United States, especially among older adults. Scientific advances have greatly reduced the likelihood of death caused by infections, allowing people to survive many years without acute illness, and experience far longer life expectancies. Such medical progress, however, has created more room for the emergence of chronic diseases such as type 2 diabetes, cardiovascular problems, arthritis, osteoporosis, obesity, muscle wasting, gum disease, dementia, and malnutrition. These conditions, among many others, place a significant burden on individuals and their caregivers, and present a distinct collection of nutrition and age-related issues.

Type 2 Diabetes

Type 2 diabetes occurs when the body cannot produce or respond normally to insulin, which is a hormone that the body needs to absorb and use blood sugar (glucose) as fuel for its cells. As a result, blood glucose levels rise abnormally and remain chronically high, leading to the development of serious and disabling complications, such as kidney damage, heart disease, impaired eye sight, **peripheral neuropathy**, and poor circulation.

Type 2 diabetes affects more than 29 million people in the United States, up from the previous estimate of 26 million in 2010 (Centers for Disease Control and Prevention 2014b). It is the seventh leading cause of death, can lower life expectancy by up to 15 years, increases the risk of heart disease by two to four times, and is the leading cause of kidney failure, lower limb amputations, and adult-onset blindness. There are effective treatments and interventions that can prevent or delay these diabetic complications; however, almost 25 percent of Americans with diabetes are undiagnosed, so many people do not obtain critical preventative care, making diabetes an immense and complex public health challenge ("Healthy People 2020 Diabetes" n.d.).

At the same time, another 86 million adults—more than one in three—have *prediabetes*, whereby their blood sugar levels are higher than normal, but not high enough be classified as type 2 diabetes. Without appropriate interventions, such as weight loss and moderate physical activity, 15 to 30 percent of this group will eventually develop type 2 diabetes within five years (Centers for Disease Control and Prevention 2014b).

Among those aged 65 and older, more than one-quarter of adults has diabetes, and the aging population is a significant contributing factor to the epidemic's expansion. In older adults, diabetes is linked to increased likelihood of institutionalization and higher mortality risk. Older diabetics have the highest rates of major lower-extremity amputation, heart attack, visual impairment, and end-stage kidney disease of any age group (Kirkman et al. 2012). In addition to heart, kidney, and nerve damage, evidence is emerging that diabetes is also associated with additional comorbidities, such as cognitive impairment and risk of bone fracture, which are both health issues of particular concern as the American population gets older ("Healthy People 2020 Diabetes" n.d.).

While there are no age-specific recommendations for the treatment of diabetes, certain considerations are important for the disease's management in older adults. Those who are physically functional, cognitively intact, and have significant life expectancy should follow dietary recommendations and blood sugar targets developed for younger adults. The goals outlined by the American Diabetes Association (ADA) for glycemic (blood sugar) control do not specifically mention age. However, the recommendation for many adults is a **glycated hemoglobin** result (also known as HbA1c) of <7 percent, but less stringent targets (8 to 9 percent) are recommended for those with limited life expectancy, advanced diabetes complications, or extensive comorbid conditions (Kirkman et al. 2012).

Heart Disease and Stroke

As previously discussed, people with diabetes are at higher risk for cardiovascular disease, including stroke. In addition to the vascular damage caused by higher than normal blood glucose levels, older individuals with type 2 diabetes tend to be overweight and physically deconditioned with central adiposity and insulin resistance, all of which promote abnormal blood cholesterol levels and the buildup of plaque in the arteries that feed blood and oxygen to the heart (Halter et al. 2014).

Heart disease is the leading cause of death in the United States, while stroke ranks as the third leading cause. Together, heart disease and stroke are among the most widespread health problems among Americans. Currently, more than one in three adults (81.1 million) live with one or more types of cardiovascular disease. The top modifiable, and therefore preventable, risk factors for heart disease and stroke are high blood pressure, high cholesterol, cigarette smoking, diabetes, poor diet, physical inactivity, overweight, and obesity ("Healthy People 2020 Heart Disease and Stroke" n.d.).

Arthritis

Arthritis, also known as **osteoarthritis**, affects one in five American adults and is the most common cause of physical disability. There are helpful interventions—often underused—that can reduce arthritis pain and functional limitations, which include increased physical activity, self-management education, and weight-loss among overweight and obese adults ("Healthy People 2020 Arthritis, Osteoporosis, and Chronic Back Conditions" n.d.).

A high body mass index (BMI) is associated with an increased risk of arthritis of the knee in older people, likely due to years of mechanical strain on weight-bearing joints. Symptoms typically appear after the age of 40. Among those age 65 and older, the prevalence of arthritis is 68 percent in women and 58 percent in men (Villareal et al. 2005).

Osteoporosis

Osteoporosis is a disease characterized by reduced bone density and strength leading to an increased risk of fractures, particularly of the hip, wrist, and spine. In the United States, an estimated 5.3 million people age 50 and older have osteoporosis, most of who are women, while about 800,000 osteoporosis sufferers are men. Experts estimate that among this age group, half of all women and as many as one in four men will have an osteoporosis-related fracture in their lifetime ("Healthy People 2020 Arthritis, Osteoporosis, and Chronic Back Conditions" n.d.).

Uncontrollable risk factors for the development of osteoporosis

- Being over age 50
- Being female
- Menopause
- Family history of osteoporosis
- Low body weight or being small and thin
- History of broken bones or height loss

Controllable risk factors

- Inadequate intake of fruits and vegetables
- Excessive intake of protein, sodium, or caffeine
- Sedentary lifestyle
- Smoking
- Drinking too much alcohol
- Excessive weight loss
- Inadequate intake of calcium

Adults over 50 require 1,200 mg of calcium per day, which is realistically obtainable from food alone, but not always. Those who need a dietary calcium supplement should aim to get the recommended daily amount from food first and supplement only if needed to make up for any shortfall. Studies have shown that there is no added benefit to taking more calcium in supplement form than is required.

- Inadequate intake of vitamin D

Supplementary vitamin D is indicated for those who are at risk for deficiency. Many calcium supplements also contain vitamin D. Certain people are at higher risk for vitamin D deficiency, including those who spend little time in the sun or those who regularly cover up when outdoors, live in nursing homes or other institutions or who are home-bound, have certain medical conditions such as Celiac disease or inflammatory bowel disease, take medicines that affect vitamin D levels such as certain anti seizure medication, and have very dark skin.

Interestingly, studies have shown that obesity is associated with increased bone mineral density and decreased osteoporosis and hip fracture in older men and women. Both body fat mass and lean body mass are directly correlated with bone mineral density, though this relationship appears to be stronger in women than in men. One reason for this difference may be that bone loss in women is partly attributed to the drop in estrogen that occurs after menopause. However, because of the increased conversion of certain compounds in adipose tissue into estrogen, the rate of bone loss is slower in postmenopausal women with higher BMIs (Villareal et al. 2005).

Higher bone density in obese individuals has also been attributed to the mechanical burden placed on weight-bearing bone tissue. However, protective effects have also been observed in nonweight-bearing bones; therefore, researchers speculate that certain hormones, such as estrogen, insulin, and leptin, are increased in people who are obese, and might contribute to the beneficial effects of obesity on bone density. These hormones are known to stimulate bone growth and inhibit bone breakdown (Villareal et al. 2005).

Sarcopenia

As adults grow older, they experience changes in body composition characterized by loss of muscle mass and strength along with a concurrent increase in fat mass—a shift called *sarcopenia*—estimated to affect about 50 percent of those older than 75. Between the ages of 30 and 70, lean body mass progressively decreases by 40 percent. At the same time, there is a rise in intra-abdominal fat along with a greater relative decrease in peripheral skeletal muscle (Villareal et al. 2005).

Sarcopenia is a complex condition believed to be driven by a combination of metabolic changes that involve fat tissue production of pro-inflammatory hormones as well as **insulin resistance**, both of which hasten muscle break down (Stenholm et al. 2008). A sedentary lifestyle and inadequate nutrient intake are also contributing factors to the development of sarcopenia, a situation that may eventually lead to malnutrition, worsening disability, functional dependence, and death (Bernstein and Munoz 2012). Although primarily a disease of the elderly, sarcopenia can also develop at any age from conditions like muscular disuse, malnutrition, and neuromuscular diseases (Merlini, Vagheggini, and Cocchi 2014).

The term *sarcopenia* comes from the Greek words sarx (meaning flesh) and penia (meaning loss) and was originally meant to represent age-related loss of muscle mass. At the time this terminology was created, scientists believed that the decline of muscle strength associated with aging was directly caused by the loss of muscle mass. However, further analysis reveals that loss of muscle strength and function can be attributed in part to the deterioration of muscle quality, such as a decrease in muscle fiber size and number, contractility of the intact fibers, level of fat infiltration into muscle, and impaired neurological regulation of muscular contraction. For these reasons, muscle strength may be more important than muscle mass as a determinant of functional limitation in older adults (Stenholm et al. 2008).

Obesity

Obesity is defined as excessive fat accumulation that negatively affects health and is indicated by a BMI of ≥ 30 kg/m^2, and a waist circumference greater than 102 cm (40 in.) in men and 88 cm (35 in.) in women. Whether these criteria are appropriate for older individuals has been questioned because of conflicting findings on the link between obesity and mortality in this population. Studies of BMI and death rates suggest that underweight is predictive of mortality, but the relationship of overweight and obesity with mortality in older adults specifically is not as clear (Bernstein and Munoz 2012).

Energy reserves during times of stress or illness, decreased risks for osteoporosis, lower likelihood of falls, and reduced postfall trauma may explain some of the observed protective effects seen in overweight or obese older adults. Other studies indicate that obesity is associated with decreased survival and lessens life expectancy, but particularly in younger adults (Bernstein and Munoz 2012; Villareal et al. 2005).

Researchers speculate that the influence of obesity on mortality may vary according to age, which may explain these discrepancies in outcome (Bernstein and Munoz 2012).

However, it is generally accepted that obesity in older adults contributes to higher risk for degenerative diseases, such as osteoarthritis, as well as age-related declines in health and physical function. Excessive calorie intake and poor food choices, in combination with physical inactivity, have resulted in a growing number of overweight and obese older adults over the last 20 years (Bernstein and Munoz 2012).

The key findings from the most recent National Health and Nutrition Examination Survey show that from 2011 to 2014, the prevalence of obesity among adults was just over 36 percent, and higher in women (38.3 percent) than in men (34.3 percent). The prevalence of obesity was higher among middle-agers 40 to 59 (40.2 percent) and older adults (37 percent) compared with younger adults 20 to 39 (32.3 percent) (National Center for Health Statisitcs 2015).

Across all adult age groups, the prevalence of obesity remains higher than the Healthy People 2020 goal of 30.5 percent. Weight loss in overweight and obese older adults has been shown to confer as much benefit as for younger adults, including lower risk of chronic disease, reduced medical complications and disability, lower mechanical burden on weak joints, and improved physical and lower extremity functioning and mobility (Bernstein and Munoz 2012).

Despite some of these positive outcomes, the benefits of weight loss among the frail elderly in particular remains unclear. Aging causes a progressive decrease in muscle mass and strength and an increase in joint dysfunction and arthritis, leading to frailty severe enough to cause disability. Frail older adults may experience severe limitations in daily activities, such as grooming, eating, bathing, shopping, and climbing stairs. Among older noninstitutionalized adults, about 20 percent of those age 65 and older, and 46 percent of those age 85 and older are considered to be frail (Villareal et al. 2005). If excess fat mass is targeted for the purpose of intentional weight loss, this can further accelerate muscle loss and exacerbate functional limitations. Therefore, careful consideration should be given to whether the benefits of weight loss outweigh the risks for certain older adults (Bernstein and Munoz 2012).

Sarcopenic Obesity

Sarcopenic obesity is the combination of two potentially disabling conditions associated with aging—sarcopenia and the significant accumulation of excess body fat. The presence of undernourished but obese older adults in a kind of nutrition paradox with added health risks. The main features of sarcopenic obesity are deterioration of muscle composition and quality in combination with increased fat mass, which results in worse physical functional declines than just sarcopenia or obesity alone (Bernstein and Munoz 2012).

Excess energy intake, physical inactivity, reduced basal metabolic rate (from muscle atrophy), low-grade inflammation, insulin resistance, and hormonal changes have all been implicated in the cause and progression of sarcopenic obesity (Bernstein and Munoz 2012). Older adults tend to obtain inadequate amounts of dietary protein, which may impair protein muscle turnover, especially during periods of weight loss. While obesity may protect against risk of death (as previously mentioned), if it exists in combination with low muscle strength, the risk of mortality may exceed the protective effect (Stenholm et al. 2008).

Dementias

Dementia is a general term for diseases and conditions involving memory loss and functional decline that interferes with daily life, and is caused by damage to the neurons in the brain. The most common type of dementia, Alzheimer's disease, currently affects approximately 5 million older adults in the United States and is the sixth leading cause of death among adults aged 18 years and older (Douglas and Lawrence 2015).

Other forms of dementia include **vascular dementia** and **Parkinson's dementia**. Because it is a progressive condition, most sufferers experience an average of four to eight years of illness and worsening decline before dying. With advancing disease, individuals lose the ability to manage many activities of daily living, including dressing, grooming, walking, and self-feeding. Many people diagnosed with Alzheimer's disease and other forms of dementia are institutionalized for care. Approximately 42 percent of older adults living in assisted living facilities and

64 percent of those living in nursing homes have some form of dementia (Douglas and Lawrence 2015).

Memory loss is a common symptom of dementia, although its manifestation does not mean a person has dementia. It is important to distinguish dementia from temporary, reversible conditions that may cause impaired cognitive functioning such as strokes, side effects from medication, chronic alcoholism, certain brain tumors and infections, vitamin B12 deficiency, and dehydration ("Healthy People 2020 Dementias, including Alzheimer's Disease" 2015).

Age and family history are among the risk factors for developing dementia. Among adults age 65 years and older, the prevalence of Alzheimer's disease doubles every five years. People with a family history of Alzheimer's disease are generally considered to be at greater risk of developing it ("Healthy People 2020 Dementias, including Alzheimer's Disease" 2015).

Because dementia leads to both physical and cognitive declines, nutritional status frequently declines as well. In the early stages of dementia, older adults may have difficulty shopping for food and preparing meals. As cognitive function continues to deteriorate, dementia sufferers may become unable to recognize and communicate feelings of hunger and thirst, or they may even forget to eat all together. These circumstances often lead to inadequate dietary intake resulting in weight loss, malnutrition, as well as increased morbidity and mortality (Douglas and Lawrence 2015).

In order to maintain adequate nutritional status and oral intake in older adults with dementia, certain studied interventions appear to improve dietary intake, such as providing finger foods, using special feeding equipment and adaptive devices to promote self-feeding, providing foods with modified textures, and offering smaller, more frequent meals. Appetite stimulants and oral liquid nutrition supplements may also improve nutrition status in this population (Douglas and Lawrence 2015).

Oral Health and Older Adults

More than ever before, older people are keeping their natural teeth. Nonetheless, serious dental problems are common among those age

65 and older, with one-third having untreated dental decay, and slightly over 40 percent suffering from **periodontal disease**. However, only 22 percent of older persons are covered by dental insurance, as many lose this type of insurance coverage after retirement, so most of their dental expenses are paid out-of-pocket (National Center for Health Statisitcs 2010).

Many older Americans grew up without the benefit of community water fluoridation and use of other products manufactured with added fluoride. Those with the poorest oral health tend to be the most economically disadvantaged, disabled, homebound, or institutionalized (Division of Oral Health 2013).

About 25 percent of adults age 60 and older no longer have any natural teeth. Having missing teeth can affect nutrition status, since their food choices may be limited to soft foods, even if they have dentures. Periodontal disease or tooth decay is the most frequent cause of tooth loss. Most older Americans take both prescription and over-the-counter drugs, and there are more than 400 commonly used medications that may significantly reduce the flow of saliva. Dry mouth increases the risk for oral disease, since saliva contains antimicrobial components and minerals that promote the rebuilding of tooth enamel attacked by decay-causing bacteria (Division of Oral Health 2013).

To maintain oral health, older adults are advised to do the following:

- Drink fluoridated water and use fluoride toothpaste; fluoride provides protection against dental decay at all ages.
- Practice good oral hygiene; careful tooth brushing and flossing to reduce dental plaque can help prevent periodontal disease.
- See a dentist regularly, even if they have no natural teeth and have dentures. Professional care helps to maintain the overall health of the teeth and mouth.
- Avoid tobacco; smokers have seven times the risk of developing periodontal disease compared to nonsmokers; tobacco used in the form of cigarettes, cigars, pipes, and spit tobacco also increases the risk for periodontal disease, oral and throat cancers, and oral fungal infections.

Source: Division of Oral Health (2013).

Malnutrition

As previously discussed, older adults often have multiple medical conditions, along with use of numerous prescription and over-the-counter medications that can impact dietary intake. In addition to these barriers to eating well, older adults also experience several physiologic changes to taste sensations and smell, along with reduced appetite—often referred to as anorexia of aging. Consequently, food intake and appetite typically decline in older adults accompanied by increased difficulties with digestion and absorption. These changes may be a direct result of aging, disease, side effect of medication use, or some combination of these factors (Bernstein and Munoz 2012). The end result is malnutrition, a significant and under-recognized problem in older adults.

The prevalence of malnutrition in older adults varies widely depending on the setting and assessment method used, but estimates range from 17 to 65 percent. Individuals residing in long-term care facilities are at greatest nutritional risk, with malnutrition more likely among older residents and those who need a higher level of care. Studies show that about one in two long-term-care residents are malnourished, which may result in increased hospital admissions and length of stay, as well as increased incidence of **pressure ulcers**, falls, and hip fractures. Rapid involuntary weight loss and low BMI in older individual often suggest underlying disease, and are often associated with poor health outcomes, deteriorating well-being, and higher mortality rates (Bernstein and Munoz 2012; Isenring et al. 2012).

For the elderly and malnourished, dietary restrictions associated with chronic diseases can compromise nutritional status even further. A prescribed diet that is too restrictive can be intolerable for older adults and contribute to poor food or fluid intake. Therefore, health care providers should carefully assess the benefits and risks associated with therapeutic diets and consider less restrictive dietary interventions that are customized to individual nutritional requirements, food preferences, and medical conditions (Bernstein and Munoz 2012).

Physical Activity

Regular physical activity and exercise are key interventions in the prevention and treatment of functional decline and frailty that occur with aging. Unfortunately, fewer than 5 percent of adults participate in 30 minutes of exercise each day, and participation in physical activity declines with age. Frailty and functional disability do not necessarily rule out exercise or regular physical activity for older adults, and often these individuals can benefit the most from a carefully planned program designed and supervised by a trained specialist (Bernstein and Munoz 2012).

Studies have shown that a combined regimen of aerobic, resistance, balance and flexibility exercises significantly decreased the risk of falls among older adults who are frail. In a randomized clinical trial, subjects with Alzheimer's dementia who participated in a home-based exercise program of **aerobic exercise** and **resistance exercise** under the supervision of their caregivers were more active and had better motor functioning compared to a control group after three months. The majority of evidence indicates that regular physical activity or exercise is beneficial to frail older adults, or those who are at high risk for frailty. The number of adverse events related to supervised physical activity has been shown to be minimal, and the gains of regular exercise clearly outweigh the risks (Liu and Fielding 2011).

For adults aged 65 and older who are generally fit and have no limiting health conditions, national guidelines call for 150 minutes of moderate-intensity aerobic activity such as brisk walking every week and muscle-strengthening activities, such as using resistance bands, lifting appropriate weights, or performing yoga exercises, on two or more days of the week that work all the major muscle group, including the legs, hips, back, abdomen, chest, shoulders, and arms.

Source: Centers for Disease Control and Prevention (2015).

Key Terms

Aerobic Exercise
Physical exercise of low to high intensity that depends primarily on the aerobic (use of oxygen) energy-generating process and intended to strengthen heart and lung function among other benefits. Examples include walking, jogging, or cycling.

Atrophic Gastritis
Bacterial overgrowth of the stomach that leads to inflammation and decreased secretion of hydrochloric acid and pepsin, which in turn impair vitamin B12 absorption.

Chronic Disease
A long-lasting condition of three months or more than can be controlled but not cured.

Epigenetics
The study of changes in organisms caused by modification of gene expression rather than alteration of the genetic code itself.

Epigenome
The collection of chemical compounds and proteins that can attach to DNA and turn genes "on" (gene expression) or turn them "off."

Fecal Impaction
Accumulation of hardened, dry feces that remains stuck in the rectum or sigmoid colon and often occurs in individuals with long-standing bowel problems or chronic constipation.

Geriatric
Relating to elderly people, especially with regard to their health care.

Glycated Hemoglobin
A protein contained inside red blood cells that binds with glucose in the blood, therefore becoming "glycated." A measurement of glycated hemoglobin offers an indication of average blood sugar levels over a period of weeks or months. For people without diabetes, a normal HbA1c range is between 4% and 5.6%. For people with diabetes, a target level is 7%.

Incontinence
Any accidental or involuntary loss of urine from the bladder or feces from the bowel.

Insulin Resistance
The diminished ability of cells to respond to the action of insulin in transporting glucose from the bloodstream into muscle and other tissues.

Intrinsic Factor
A protein produced by the stomach that is needed to absorb vitamin B12 in the intestine.

Life Span
The length of life for an organism.

Longevity
Great duration of individual life.

Megaloblastic Anemia
A disorder in which red blood cells are immature, larger than normal, and few in number, reducing the amount of oxygen that can be carried by the blood to the body's tissues.

Morbidity
How often a disease occurs; the incidence of a disease, as a rate of a population, which is affected; adverse effects caused by a medical treatment such as surgery or radiation therapy.

Mortality
The death rate, which reflects the number of deaths per unit of population in any specific region, age group, disease, or other classification.

Osteoarthritis
Also known as degenerative joint disease; a form of arthritis in which the protective cartilage on the ends of bones wears down over time and commonly affects joints in the hands, knees, hips, and spine leading to pain, stiffness, and swelling.

Parkinson's Dementia
A form of dementia associated with the advanced stages of Parkinson's disease—a degenerative neurological disorder resulting from insufficient production of the brain chemical dopamine.

Periodontal Disease
A bacterial infection caused by the buildup of plaque that destroys the fibers and supporting bones that support the teeth. Left untreated, it can lead to tooth loss.

Peripheral Neuropathy

A condition in which there is damage to the peripheral nerves, often causing weakness, numbness, and pain typically in the hands and feet.

Pernicious Anemia

An autoimmune disease that impairs the body's ability to make intrinsic factor.

Pressure Ulcer

A localized injury to the skin or underlying tissue usually over a bony prominence as a result of pressure and shear, often from being malnourished and bedridden. The ulcers or sores can range from being mildly red to producing severe muscle and bone damage, as well as life-threatening infections.

Resistance Exercise

Any exercise that causes the muscles to contract against an external resistance with the aim of increasing strength, tone, mass, and endurance. Examples include lifting free weights, using weight machines or stretchy resistance bands, or using one's own body weight.

Successful Aging

Physical, mental, and social well-being in older age.

Vascular Dementia

A form of dementia caused by impaired supply of blood to the brain. May be caused by small strokes or other conditions that damage blood vessels. Risk factors include high blood pressure, high cholesterol, and smoking.

References

Bernstein, M., and N. Munoz. August 2012. "Position of the Academy of Nutrition and Dietetics: Food and Nutrition for Older Adults: Promoting Health and Wellness." *Journal of the Academy of Nutrition and Dietetics* 112, no. 8, pp. 1255–77.

Centers for Disease Control and Prevention. 2014a. "Leading Causes of Deaths, By Age: United States, 1980 and 2013." www.cdc.gov/nchs/data/hus/2014/021.pdf

Centers for Disease Control and Prevention. June 10, 2014b. "More Than 29 Million Americans Have Diabetes; 1 in 4 Doesn't Know." www.cdc.gov/media/releases/2014/p0610-diabetes-report.html

Centers for Disease Control and Prevention. June 4, 2015. "How Much Physical Activity Do Older People Need?" www.cdc.gov/physicalactivity/basics/older_adults/

Division of Oral Health. July 10, 2013. "Oral Health for Older Americans." Centers for Disease Control and Prevention. www.cdc.gov/oralhealth/publications/factsheets/adult_oral_health/adult_older.htm (accessed November 15, 2015).

Douglas, J.W., and J.C. Lawrence. November 2015. "Environmental Considerations for Improving Nutritional Status in Older Adults with Dementia: A Narrative Review." *Journal of the Academy of Nutrition and Dietetics* 115, no. 11, pp. 1815–31.

Evans, C.J., Y. Ho, B.A. Daveson, S. Hall, I.J. Higginson, and W. Gao. 2014. "Place and Cause of Death in Centenarians: A Population-Based Observational Study in England, 2001 to 2010." *PLoS Medicine* 11, no. 6.

Halter, J.B., N. Musi, F.M. Horne, J.P. Crandall, A. Goldberg, L. Harkless, W.R. Hazzard, E.S. Huang, M.S. Kirkman, J. Plutzky, and K.E. Schmader. August 2014. "Diabetes and Cardiovascular Disease in Older Adults: Current Status and Future Directions." *Diabetes* 63, no. 8, pp. 2578–89.

"Healthy People 2020 Arthritis, Osteoporosis, and Chronic Back Conditions." n.d. U.S. Department of Health and Human Services. Office of Disease Prevention and Health Promotion. www/healthypeople.gov/2020/topics-objectives/topic/Arthritis-Osteoporosis-and-Chronic-Back-Conditions (accessed November 15, 2015).

"Healthy People 2020 Dementias, including Alzheimer's Disease." n.d. Office of Disease Prevention and Health Promotion. U.S. Department of Health and Human Services. www.healthypeople.gov/2020/topics-objectives/topic/dementias-including-alzheimers-disease (accessed November 15, 2015).

"Healthy People 2020 Diabetes." n.d. U.S. Department of Health and Human Services. Office of Disease Prevention and Health promotion. www.healthypeople.gov/2020/topics-objectives/topic/diabetes (accessed November 15, 2015).

"Healthy People 2020 Heart Disease and Stroke." n.d. U.S. Department of Health and Human Services. Office of Disease Prevention and Health Promotion. www.healthypeople.gov/2020/topics-objectives/topic/heart-disease-and-stroke (accessed November 15, 2015).

"Healthy People 2020 Older Adults." n.d. U.S. Department of Health and Human Services. Office of Disease Prevention and Health Promotion. www.healthypeople.gov/2020/topics-objectives/topic/older-adults. (accessed November 15, 2015).

Isenring, E.A., M. Banks, M. Ferguson, and J.D. Bauer. March 2012. "Beyond Malnutrition Screening: Appropriate Methods to Guide Nutrition Care for Aged Care Residents." *Journal of the American Academy of Nutrition and Dietetics* 112, no. 3, pp. 376–81.

Kirkman, M.S., V.J. Briscoe, N. Clark, H. Florez, L.B. Haas, J.B. Halter, E.S. Huang, M.T. Korytkowski, M.N. Munshi, P.S. Odegard, and R.E. Pratley. December 2012. "Diabetes in Older Adults." *Diabetes Care* 35, no. 12, pp. 2650–64.

Liu, C.K., and R.A. Fielding. February 2011. "Exercise as an Intervention for Frailty." *Clinics in Geriatric Medicine* 27, no. 1, pp. 101–10.

Merlini, L., A. Vagheggini, and D. Cocchi. 2014. "Sarcopenia and Sarcopenic Obesity in Patients with Muscular Dystrophy." *Frontiers in Aging Neuroscience* 6, no. 274.

Mozaffarian, D., and D.S. Ludwig. June 2015. "The 2015 US Dietary Guidelines. Lifting the Ban on Total Dietary Fat." *Journal of the American Medical Association* 313, no. 24, pp. 2421–22.

National Center for Health Statistics. January 26, 2010. "Health of Older Americans." Centers for Disease Control and Prevention. www.cdc.gov/nchs/pressroom/01facts/olderame.htm (accessed November 15, 2015).

National Center for Health Statistics. November 20, 2015. "Prevalence of Obesity Among Adults and Youth: United States, 2011–2014." U.S. Department of Health and Human Services. www.cdc.gov/nchs/data/databriefs/db219.pdf

National Institute on Aging. November 2011. "Biology of Aging: Research Today for a Healthier Tomorrow." National Institutes of Health. U.S. Department of Health and Human Services. www.nia.nih.gov/health/publication/biology-aging (accessed November 3, 2015).

National Institutes of Health. November 2014. "Eating Well As You Get Older." www.nihseniorhealth.gov/eatingwellasyougetolder/knowhowmuchtoeat/01.html

Stenholm, S., T.B. Harris, T. Rantanen, M. Visser, S.B. Kritchevsky, and L. Ferrucci. November 2008. "Sarcopenic Obesity: Definition, Cause and Consequences." *Current Opinion in Clinical Nutrition and Metabolic Care* 11, no. 6, pp. 693–700.

Thomas, J., C.J. Thomas, J. Radcliffe, and C. Itsiopoulos. 2015. "Omega-3 Fatty Acids in Early Prevention of Inflammatory Neurodegenerative Disease: A Focus on Alzheimer's Disease." *BioMed Research International* 2015: 172801.

U.S. Census Bureau, Population Estimates. 2013. http://factfinder.census.gov/bkmk/table/1.0/en/PEP/2013/PEPAGESEX

U.S. Census Bureau, Population Estimates. 2014. Population Projections. www. census.gov/population/projections/data/national/2014/

Villareal, D.T., C.M. Apovian, R.F. Kushner, and S. Klein. November 2005. "Obesity in Older Adults: Technical Review and Position Statement of the American Society for Nutrition and NAASO, The Obesity Society." *The American Journal of Clinical Nutrition* 82, no. 5, pp. 923–34.

Additional Resources

The work presented here is a summary of how nutrient and energy requirements change throughout the human lifecycle and affect long-term health. While many details were included, the information in this text is by no means exhaustive—there is much to know about age-appropriate dietary needs and interventions, and scientific research continues to reveal new insights.

For additional information, the following resources may be helpful:

March of Dimes Birth Defect Foundation
www.marchofdimes.com

International Lactation Consultant Association
www.ilca.org

La Leche League International
www.llli.org

Women, Infants, and Children (WIC)
www.fns.usda.gov/wic/women-infants-and-children-wic

Choose My Plate for Children
www.choosemyplate.gov/children

Center for Adolescent Health, Johns Hopkins Bloomberg School of Public Health
www.jhsph.edu/research/centers-and-institutes/center-for-adolescent-health/

Administration on Aging (AoA)
www.aoa.gov

NIH Senior Health
www.nihseniorhealth.gov

Index

ACOG. *See* American College of Obstetricians and Gynecologists (ACOG)
active transport, 31
adipose tissue, 33
adiposity, 80
adolescents
　alcohol, smoking and drug use, 104–109
　athletic teen, 112–114
　body image, 114–115
　calcium, 102–103
　carbohydrates, 101
　daily serving recommendations, 99–104, 100*t*
　disordered eating *versus* eating disorder, 115–116
　drug use, 107–109
　energy, 99, 101
　fats, 102
　growth, 97–98, 83
　iron, 104
　key features in, 98*t*
　nutrition for, 97–119
　nutrient requirements, 99
　obesity, 109–112
　overview, 97
　pregnancy, 45–46
　protein, 101–102
　risk factors for osteoporosis, 103
　smoking, 106–107
　vitamin D, 102–103
adolescents obesity, 109–112
　factors influencing, 111
　health risks and, 111–112
　treatment and interventions, 112
aerobic exercise, 93, 142
ALA. *See* alpha-linolenic acid
alcohol
　adolescents, 104–106
　during pregnancy, 45
　related risks, 106

allergenic, 70
alpha-linolenic acid (ALA), 14, 17*t*
Alzheimer's disease, 139
amenorrhea, 3
American College of Obstetricians and Gynecologists (ACOG), 32
anabolic steroids, 116
anthropometric measure, 80
antiemetics, 43
athletic teen, 112–114
　energy, 112–113
　fluids, 113
　macronutrients, 113–114
　micronutrients, 114
atopic dermatitis, 67
atrophic gastritis, 129

basal metabolic rate (BMR), 83
binge drinking, 105
bioavailability, 104
bioelectrical impedance, 80
BMI. *See* body mass index
BMR. *See* basal metabolic rate
body image, 80
　adolescents, 114–115
　in early and middle childhood, 80
beta-carotene, 5
blastocyst, 28
body mass index (BMI), 3, 32, 80–82
　2 to 20 years: boys, 81*f*
　2 to 20 years: girls, 82*f*
　interpreting, 82–83
bone mineralization, 7
bone-strengthening activities, 93
breastfeeding, 63–68
　benefits of, 66–67
　contraindications to, 67–68
　maternal diet and, 67–68
　physiology of breast milk production, 64–66
Bulimia Nervosa, 115

calcium, 9–11, 10*t*–11*t*, 41
  adolescents, 102–103
  infant, feeding, 61
  older adults, 129
carbohydrate
  adolescents, 101
  during pregnancy, 37–38
  early and middle childhood, 84
  infant, feeding, 56–57
  older adults, 127
carotenoids, 5
casein, 69
Centers for Disease Control and
        Prevention (CDC), 54, 110
  prevention checklist, 18–19
cesarean delivery, 3
changing demographics in older
        adults, 121–123
childhood obesity, 91–93
choline, 40
Choose My Plate website, 86, 99, 127
chronic disease, 122
  impact on older adults, 131–139
    arthritis, 133
    dementia, 138–139
    heart disease and stroke, 133
    obesity, 136–137
    osteoporosis, 133–135
    sarcopenia, 135–136
    sarcopenic obesity, 138
    type 2 diabetes, 131–132
cilia, 28
cognitive development, 104
cognitive function, 40
colostrum, 65
complementary foods, infant, 70–74
  balanced variety of foods, 72
  behavioral signs, 70
  foods to avoid, 73–74
  standard milk-based infant
        formulas and breast milk, 71*t*
conception, 1
congenital heart problems, 3
constipation, 43–44
corpus luteum, 28

Daily Food Plans, 86, 99
daily serving recommendations
  adolescents, 99–104, 100*t*

early and middle childhood, 86–88,
        87*t*
  older adults, 126–129, 126*t*
dementia, 138–139
developmental milestones, 83
developmental programming, x
Dietary Reference Intake (DRI), 34,
        35*t*–36*t*, 55, 129
The Dietary Guidelines for Americans,
        ix
disordered eating *versus* eating
        disorder, 115–116
diuretic, 115
docosahexaenonic acid (DHA), 14
dopamine, 108
DRI. *See* Dietary Reference Intake
drug use
  adolescents, 107–109
  during pregnancy, 45

early and middle childhood, 79–95
  carbohydrates, 84
  childhood obesity, 91–93
  daily serving recommendations,
        86–88, 87*t*
  fats, 85
  food safety and, 89
  growth and body mass index,
        80–82
  Healthy People 2020, 88
  nutrient requirements, 83–85
  oral health, 89–91
  overview, 79
  protein, 83–84
  vitamins and minerals, 85–86
ectopic pregnancy, 28
EER. *See* Estimated Energy
        Requirements
EFA. *See* essential fatty acids
eicosapentaenoic acid (EPA), 14
electrolytes, 113
embryo, 2
endocytosis, 31
endometrium, 28
energy needs, 37
  adolescents, 99, 101
  athletic teen, 112–113
  infant, feeding, 56
  older adults, 125–126

Environmental Protection Agency
    (EPA), 14
epididymitis, 17
epigenetics, 130
epigenome, 130
epithelial tissue, 5
essential fatty acids (EFA), 14–17,
    15t–16t
Estimated Energy Requirements
    (EER), 55
estrogen, 28

fallopian tube, 28
facilitated diffusion, 31
failure to thrive, 59
fat
    adolescents, 102
    early and middle childhood, 85
    for fetal growth, 38–39
    older adults, 128
fatty liver disease, 92
FDA. See Food and Drug
    Administration
fecal impaction, 127
feeding, infant, 53–75
fetal alcohol syndrome, 45
fetal development, 28–30
    stages of, 29t–30t
fetal placenta, 30
fetus, 1, 29
fluids
    athletic teen, 113
    older adults, 126–127
fluoride, infant feeding, 62
fluorosis, 62
folate
    during pregnancy, 39
    infant, feeding, 60
    preconception nutrition, 7, 8t
folic acid, 39
Food and Drug Administration
    (FDA), 14, 39
food safety, 44–45
    during pregnancy, 44–45
    young children and, 89
foodborne illness, 44
foremilk, 65

gene expression, 1
genetic reprogramming, 4
geriatric certification, 123
gestation, 1
gestational diabetes, 3, 42–43
gestational hypertension and
    preeclampsia, 41–42
gluconeogenesis, 113
glycated hemoglobin, 4, 132
growth
    of adolesents, 97–98
    of early and middle childhood,
        80–82
    of infant, 53–55
growth velocity, 80

heart disease, ix, 133
heartburn, 43–44
hindmilk, 65
hippocampus, 105
human chorionic gonadotropin
    (hCG), 28
human placental lactogen (hPL), 31
hydrolyzed, 70
hyperemesis gravidarum, 43

immunological factors, 67
implantation, 2
incontinence, fear of, 126
infant reflexes, 55
infant formula, 68–69
    lactose-intolerance in, 69
    soy-based, 69
    types of, 69–70
infant, feeding, 53–75
    breastfeeding, 63–68
    calcium, 61
    complementary foods, 70–74
    fluoride, 62
    folate, 60
    growth, 53–55
    infant formula, 68–69
    iron, 60–61
    nutrient requirements, 55–63
        carbohydrates, 56–57
        energy, 56
        fats, 57–58

protein, 57
vitamins and minerals, 58–63
overview, 53
reflexes, 55
vitamin A, 59
vitamin B12, 59–60
vitamin C, 59
water, 62–63
zinc, 61–62
infant mortality, ix
infertility, 3
Institute of Medicine (IOM), 10, 32, 129
Food and Nutrition Board, 55
insulin, 42
intrauterine growth restriction, 12–13, 33
intrinsic factor, 129
iodine, 11, 12t, 41
IOM. *See* Institute of Medicine
iron, 11–14, 13t–14t, 40–41
adolescents, 104
infant, feeding, 60–61
iron-deficiency anemia, 43

labor, third stage of, 31
lactation, 31
laxative, 115
lean body mass, 92
let-down reflex, 65
life span, 121
longevity, understanding, 129–131

macronutrients, 113–114
macrosomia, 4
malnutrition in older adults, 141
mammary glands, 64
maternal diet, breastfeeding and, 67–68
maternal nutrition, 4–5
maternal placenta, 30
meconium, 53
megaloblastic anemia, 60, 129
men
CDC prevention checklist, 18–19
weight and nutrition for, 17–18
metabolic syndrome, 92

micronutrients, 114
milk ejection reflex, 65
morbidity, 130
mortality, 124
muscle-strengthening activities, 93
MyPlate for Older Adults, 124

National Survey on Drug Use and Health (NSDUH), 105
neonatal death, 3
neural tube defect, 3
neurological changes in adolescents, 97
neuroplasticity, 108
nicotine, 106
nutrition for healthy pregnancy, 27–49
overview, 27–28
neonatal death, 32
nutrient requirements
adolescents, 99
during pregnancy, 34–41
carbohydrate, 37–38
energy, 37
fat, 38–39
protein, 38
vitamins and minerals, 39–41
early and middle childhood, 83–85
infant, feeding, 55–63
obesity, ix
osteoporosis, 3

obesity
defined, 110
in older adults, 136–137
sarcopenic, 138
obesogenic diet, 92
older adults, 121–145
calcium, 129
carbohydrate, 127
changing demographics, 121–123
daily serving recommendations, 126–129, 126t
energy needs, 125–126
fats, 128
fluids, 126–127
impact of chronic disease, 131–139

malnutrition, 141
nutrition and health promotion, 123–124
oral health and, 139–140
overview, 121
physical activity, 141–142
protein, 127–128
understanding longevity, 129–131
vitamin B12, 128–129
vitamin D, 129
omega-3 docosahexaenonic acid (DHA), 70
omega-6 arachidonic acid (ARA), 70
oral health
early and middle childhood, 89–91
older adults and, 139–140
osteoarthritis, 91, 112, 133
osteoporosis, 103, 133–135
risk factors for, 103, 134
oxytocin, 64

Parkinson's dementia, 138
passive diffusion, 31
paternal health, 17–23
weight and nutrition for men, 17–18
peak bone mass, 103
periconceptional period, 2
periodontal disease, 140
peripheral neuropathy, 131
peristalsis, 28
pernicious anemia, 129
Physical Activity Guidelines for Americans, 93
physical activity in older adults, 141–142
placenta, 2, 30–32
fetal, 30
maternal, 30
placental abruption, 45
postpartum, 65
potassium, 113
preconception care, 1, 3t
preconception nutrition, 1–23
overview, 1
paternal health, 17–23
preparing for pregnancy, 1–17

prediabetes, 91
preeclampsia, 3
prefrontal cortex, 108
pregestational diabetes, 4
pregnancy
nutrition for healthy, 27–49
adolescent pregnancy, 45–46
constipation and heartburn, 43–44
fetal development, 28–30
food safety, 44–45
gestational diabetes, 42–43
gestational hypertension and preeclampsia, 41–42
hyperemesis gravidarum, 43
iron-deficiency anemia, 43
placenta, 30–32
prenatal supplements, 44
smoking, alcohol, and drugs, 45
weight gain during pregnancy, 32–33, 33t
preparing for, 1–17
calcium, 9–11, 10t–11t
essential fatty acids (EFA), 14–17, 15t–16t
folate, 7, 8t
iodine, 11, 12t
maternal nutrition, 4–5
multivitamin supplements, 5
pregestational diabetes, 4
vitamin A, 5–7, 6t
vitamin D, 7, 9, 9t
weight, 3–4
prenatal supplements, 44
pressure ulcers, 141
prolactin, 64
protein, 38
adolescents, 101–102
early and middle childhood, 83–84
infant, feeding, 57
older adults, 127–128
preterm birth, 3
progesterone, 28
puberty, 83

recumbent length, 54
relaxin, 31

renal solute load, 63
resistance exercise, 142
retinoids, 5

sarcopenia, 135–136
sarcopenic obesity, 138
secondary sexual characteristics, 97
shoulder dystocia, 32
skinfold thickness, 80
sleep apnea, 111
small-for-gestational-age newborns, 3
smoking
    in adolescents, 106–107
    during pregnancy, 45
sodium, 113
stem cell, 40
stigmatization, 111
stillbirths, 3
stimulant, 106
stroke, 133
successful aging, 123

teratogenic effects, 2
tubal pregnancy, 28
type 2 diabetes, ix, 131–132

umbilical cord, 31

varicoceles, 17
vascular dementia, 138
vitamins and minerals
    early and middle childhood, 85–86
vitamin A
    for healthy pregnancy, 39–40
    infant, feeding, 59
    preconception nutrition, 5–7, 6t
vitamin B12
    infant, feeding, 59–60
    older adults, 128–129
vitamin C
    infant, feeding, 59
vitamin D, 40
    adolescents, 102–103
    for healthy pregnancy, 40
    infant, feeding, 58
    older adults, 129
    preconception nutrition, 7, 9, 9t

water, feeding the infant, 62–63
weight, 3–4
    distribution, 33–34, 34t
    gain, infant, 66
    gain during pregnancy, 32–33, 33t

zinc, feeding the infant, 61–62
zygote, 28

OTHER TITLES IN OUR NUTRITION AND DIETETICS PRACTICE COLLECTION

Katie Ferraro, University of San Francisco School of Nursing, Editor

Nutrition Support
by Brenda O'Day

*Diet and Disease: Nutrition for Heart Disease,
Diabetes, and Metabolic Stress*
by Katie Ferraro

*Diet and Disease: Nutrition for Gastrointestinal, Musculoskeletal,
Hepatobiliary, Pancreatic, and Kidney Diseases*
by Katie Ferraro

Weight Management and Obesity
by Courtney Winston Paolicelli

Dietary Supplements
by B. Bryan Haycock and Amy A. Sunderman

Introduction to Dietetic Practice
by Katie Ferraro

Sports Nutrition
by Kary Woodruff

Momentum Press is one of the leading book publishers in the field of engineering, mathematics, health, and applied sciences. Momentum Press offers over 30 collections, including Aerospace, Biomedical, Civil, Environmental, Nanomaterials, Geotechnical, and many others.

Momentum Press is actively seeking collection editors as well as authors. For more information about becoming an MP author or collection editor, please visit http://www.momentumpress.net/contact

Announcing Digital Content Crafted by Librarians

Momentum Press offers digital content as authoritative treatments of advanced engineering topics by leaders in their field. Hosted on ebrary, MP provides practitioners, researchers, faculty, and students in engineering, science, and industry with innovative electronic content in sensors and controls engineering, advanced energy engineering, manufacturing, and materials science.

Momentum Press offers library-friendly terms:

- perpetual access for a one-time fee
- no subscriptions or access fees required
- unlimited concurrent usage permitted
- downloadable PDFs provided
- free MARC records included
- free trials

The **Momentum Press** digital library is very affordable, with no obligation to buy in future years.

For more information, please visit **www.momentumpress.net/library** or to set up a trial in the US, please contact **mpsales@globalepress.com**.

CPSIA information can be obtained
at www.ICGtesting.com
Printed in the USA
FFOW02n1308280217
32956FF